Coping with Phob

Professor Kevin Gournay, CBE, is an Emeritus Professor at the institute of Psychiatry (King's College London). In his clinical work at the Priory Hospital, North London, he treats phobias, panic and other anxiety disorders including post-traumatic stress disorder and obsessive–compulsive disorder. He has also worked in areas of general medicine, including cancer, cardiovascular disorders, multiple sclerosis and pain management for a number of disorders. He has managed research and training projects in the UK and across the world, and currently works part time as a consultant to the World Health Organization. He has written extensively. He has a number of national and international honours, awards and honorary degrees. He was appointed CBE in 1998–9. He also works as an expert witness in the UK and Ireland.

He is president and founding patron of No Panic, as well as being a patron and adviser to several other charities. He is a frequent contributor to TV, radio and newspapers.

Kevin is a season ticket holder and a supporter for 50 plus years of Charlton Athletic. He is a veteran of 14 marathons and is an active member of Broxbourne Runners. He lives in Hertfordshire and has four children.

Overcoming Common Problems Series

Selected titles

A full list of titles is available from Sheldon Press,
36 Causton Street, London SW1P 4ST and on our website at
www.sheldonpress.co.uk

Overcoming Common Problems

Coping with Phobias and Panic

PROFESSOR KEVIN GOURNAY

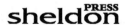

For Siobhan, Alex, Sam and Franki

First published in Great Britain in 2010

Sheldon Press
36 Causton Street
London SW1P 4ST

British Library Cataloguing-in-Publication Data
A catalogue record for this book is available from the British Library

ISBN 978-1-84709-079-9

1 3 5 7 9 10 8 6 4 2

Typeset by Fakenham Photosetting Ltd, Fakenham, Norfolk
Printed in Great Britain by Ashford Colour Press

Produced on paper from sustainable forests

Contents

Acknowledgements

I must here mention some of the people who have influenced me most in my career and who have, at various times, helped me to acquire the skills and knowledge I have today.

Professor Isaac Marks was originally my teacher at the Maudsley Hospital in the 1970s, and is, perhaps, the world's best-known authority on fears and phobias. During his academic career, he ran or supervised numerous research projects on fears and phobias and has published hundreds of books, chapters and papers. In his clinical work, Professor Marks has helped literally thousands of people. Of most relevance to the readers of this book, however, are two areas in which he has led where countless others now follow. He was the first person to recognize that the skills (of therapists) in effective psychological treatments need painstaking attention and they cannot learn all the therapy skills they need in a ten-day course or even a part-time two-year university course. Professor Marks recognized that expert therapists need literally hundreds of hours of training and an enormous amount of clinical practice – with adequate supervision. He also recognized, however, that it is not necessary to have a PhD in psychology to acquire these skills – mental health nurses and, indeed, many others, including those with no background as health professionals, can be taught to be expert therapists. Thus, many of the ideas developed by Isaac Marks some 35 years ago are now expressed in a wide range of training programmes across the Western world. It is very important to emphasize, however, that Professor Marks also realized at a very early point that 'expert' therapy is perhaps necessary only in a minority of cases and many of the commoner and relatively straightforward states of anxiety can be treated with much simpler interventions.

Within this context, Professor Marks wrote what is, within the self-help movement, a legendary book, *Living with Fear*, first published in 1978. In the last 15 years or so, Professor Marks has been at the forefront of developing computer-based self-help treatments for a range of anxiety problems. The computer program closest to his heart is Fearfighter, now recommended by the government as a first-line treatment for fears and phobias. I am sure that it is Professor Marks, along with Colin Hammond, to whom I refer below, who have been the central inspirational figures in my own efforts to promote self-help as an effective treatment.

With regard to Colin Hammond, I have known him since 1982, my initial contact with him being as his therapist. I want to make it clear that I am not breaching patient confidentiality here; Colin and I have, on many occasions, publicly told the story of his treatment to illustrate the benefits of professional treatments and the need for self-help. As Colin would, I am sure, say, his own case serves to exemplify how limited professional treatment can be and how much can be achieved by helping yourself in a structured and systematic way.

My association with No Panic, the charity that Colin founded and managed as its chief executive, began in 1991. It was Colin who suggested that I write my first self-help book on anxiety disorders and has continued to encourage me to write more – hence this book, too! Colin is now recognized as one of the leading lights of the self-help movement and I am proud to say that the charity he founded has won numerous national awards, including the Queen's Award for Voluntary Service 2004 and the Guardian Charity of the Year Award 2003. Colin himself was honoured by the Queen with an MBE three years ago.

While my primary allegiance is, of course, to No Panic, I also need to say that all the other self-help charities, past and present, should be commended for their continuing efforts. There are many different ways to deliver self-help; each of the other charities I know possesses unique individual characteristics and sometimes stark differences from its counterparts. I am grateful for this opportunity to provide my heartfelt commendation to all of those people who give huge amounts of time to the running of self-help groups and organizations.

There is a huge number of people to whom I owe debts of gratitude and I did actually write several lists before beginning this book. I would finish each list and then, shortly after, remember another name and a reason for including him or her. To avoid leaving someone out, I tore up the last such list and so simply wish to say here to all of you, an enormous 'Thank you' from myself and all of the people you have helped.

Preface

At the time of writing this book, I have been involved in treating phobias, panic and other anxiety states for nearly 35 years. For almost as many years, I have also been involved in research into the nature and treatment of these disorders. During this time I have been fortunate enough to travel across the world and meet many of the leading experts in the fields of research and treatment of anxiety and related disorders. I have also had the great pleasure, in the UK, to work with doctors, psychologists, nurses and others who have dedicated their lives to the treatment of people with anxiety disorders. I have, I hope, learned many lessons from these inspiring people and from my own research. The most important lessons, however, have come from my contact with those who themselves experience anxiety states. At the same time, one of the most salutary findings of my research and clinical experience, with several thousand people, is that professional treatment often promises much more than it delivers.

Despite the very encouraging results from research studies and an enormous increase in skill among the workforce over the past 30 years, many people with anxiety achieve only limited benefit from professional treatment. Indeed, I would go so far as to say that some people with anxiety disorders remain the same or, sadly, are worse after receiving professional treatment. Equally, I am continually surprised by the way in which people help themselves. I can think of many cases where people have abandoned years of professional treatment to 'go it alone' and have succeeded where professionals have failed.

In the 18 years or so that I have been involved in the charity No Panic, of which I am a patron and very proud president, I have been increasingly convinced that the self-help movement has a great deal to offer. Rather than seeing self-help and professional treatments as separate entities, I believe that the way forward is to obtain a blend of these two approaches. Indeed, much of the time, my own professional treatment involves helping people to help themselves.

As this book will I hope show, self-help comes in many shapes and forms, ranging from Internet-based programmes, available across the English-speaking world, to two or three people getting together over a cup of coffee or sharing their experiences on the telephone.

Self-help is not for everyone, though, so the starting point for anyone trying to help people with anxiety disorders should be to obtain the views of the people concerned as to what they think is needed. My advice in this respect is to listen to what they say; they are often the experts on themselves.

Introduction

'Fear is normal.' I probably use these three words every time I see a new client who comes to me with phobic anxiety or panic. The problem with fear is that, as with many normal phenomena, it can simply get out of hand. Fear can grow into a phobia, so that the presence of a particular object or being in a particular situation leads to a level of fear that is unpleasant and overwhelming and makes you want to escape from it at the earliest possible opportunity. Likewise, 'nervousness', which everyone feels on some occasions, can grow to such an extent that we become overwhelmed by a mixture of physical feelings and thoughts of such intensity that we feel like a catastrophe is about to occur. That catastrophic feeling may signal, to the individual concerned, that death is imminent, humiliation is inevitable or a loss of control and madness will develop, without any hope of recovery.

Fear is an essential part of all our lives. If you think about it, people *without* fear would be killed the first time they crossed a road. Ask yourself: 'Is it normal to have some fear and apprehension?' If the choice is walking down a well-lit road or taking a shortcut through a dark underpass late at night, what stops us choosing the riskier route? Is it normal to have some apprehension when walking through the undergrowth in a forest or to have butterflies in the tummy when about to ski down a glacier? Is it normal to have some apprehension about a medical check-up? All these situations involve fear. The answer to the questions, then, is 'Yes'. Indeed, if someone was to answer 'No' to any of those questions, that would be very abnormal.

Fear has a survival function: it protects us from making unwise choices and walking through the dark underpass instead of the well-lit road. Fear also protects us in a physical sense. The hormone of fear – adrenaline – prepares our body for 'fight or flight' responses to situations.

Human beings, however, are strange! Some people seem to enjoy fear. What about people who get a kick out of being scared stiff when taking a rollercoaster ride? Therein lies an interesting point. The phrase 'scared stiff' derives from the physical experience of having very tense muscles as a result of the outpouring of adrenaline – the hormone of fear – into the body. For the thrillseeker at a fairground, that tension is exactly the same physical sensation as the person who is in a chronic state of anxiety and worry and whose neck and shoulders are stiff, but their feelings about those sensations are entirely different. Fear is therefore a double-edged sword and some people seem to have more fear than others.

This is a book about phobias and panic and, as I will explain below, I deal with these two topics together as they are often inextricably linked. The majority of people I see in outpatient clinics with phobias experience panic attacks and the pattern of their panic can become as much of a problem as the phobia.

When writing this book, I had two principal aims. First, I wished to set out information about these topics and, therefore, empower those experiencing these disorders with knowledge. In my experience this is usually of central importance, as people often feel they are completely alone, when the reality is that huge numbers of people have irrational fears and states of anxiety. Information about phobias and panic is important because many people who come to me for treatment tell me that their worst, deep-down fear is that their condition will lead to madness or a breakdown. I hope that my book will assist in putting across the message that, while some phobias can be truly debilitating and at times seem overwhelming in intensity, phobias and anxieties do not develop into major mental illnesses, such as schizophrenia. Madness is never a consequence of phobias and, most important of all, for the vast majority of people there can be great levels of improvement – even a total disappearance of these symptoms is a real probability. To achieve such alleviation of suffering does not necessarily mean that you need to go to a psychiatrist, psychologist or specialist therapist; often substantial improvement can follow from self-help techniques. Indeed, there is now a huge amount of research evidence that testifies to this.

The second aim of this book is to provide practical advice about how to conquer phobias and panic. As much as I can, I have tried to use plain English as I believe that if there is a need to resort to medical jargon or unintelligible scientific terminology, there is something wrong with the message you are trying to transmit!

The book is divided into two main parts. Part 1 – Phobias and panic: the facts – sets out all you need to know about phobias and panic. I describe the commonly occurring phobias, panic and a number of conditions that also often trouble people. I say something about how it is thought phobias and panic are caused and then describe the various treatment approaches, including the roles of self-help methods and organizations.

In Part 2, I describe a tried and tested self-help programme, which I designed more than 15 years ago. The programme has been modified over time as I have learned a great deal from those who have used it and provided me with very valuable feedback.

I make no apology for emphasizing the word 'exposure'. This word is repeated in all sections of the book as exposure is the central method for conquering phobias and panic. To remove phobic fears from your life, you need to face them and Part 2 of this book teaches you how to do that.

There is an emphasis on two principles. First, exposure to phobias and panic needs to be carried out in steps, with you gradually increasing your efforts. Second, exposure should be at a level that you find difficult, but manageable. If you try to push yourself too far, you will suffer setbacks.

I must emphasize that this book will not have all the answers. I do hope, however, that, in helping you to help yourself, I can, at the very least, point you in the right direction.

A note on the case studies

The case studies and examples in this book are all based on real people. Some people have given their permission for their stories to be included, while, in other cases, details have been changed to protect their anonymity.

A note on the NICE guidelines

Throughout this book I refer to the NICE guidelines. NICE (the National Institute for Health and Clinical Excellence) is an independent organization set up by the government in the UK to be responsible for providing national guidance on promoting good health and preventing ill health. NICE has several functions, one of them being the production of clinical guidelines.

The clinical guidelines are recommendations by NICE on the appropriate care and treatment of people with specific diseases and conditions within the NHS. They are based on the best available evidence. The guidelines help health professionals in their work, but they do not replace their knowledge and skills.

The guidelines are very important as they tell you about what are considered to be the best treatments to which you are entitled. They give you not only summaries in plain English but also, for those who wish to have more information, detailed technical background.

NICE also provides a free newsletter – just visit the NICE website (at <www.nice.org.uk>) and register. The NICE website also contains details of guidelines under development.

Once a NICE guideline has been published, it becomes subject to another review after five years. The guidelines are revisited and, as necessary, amended and/or rewritten.

Part 1
PHOBIAS AND PANIC: THE FACTS

1

Categories of anxiety states

Phobias and panic are anxiety states. It is essential here to say something about how anxiety states are classified.

Anxiety states may be classified in many different ways and even professionals use different ones. In practice, however, the list that follows probably represents a reasonable general way of categorizing the various anxiety states:

- simple (specific) phobias
- social phobia or social anxiety disorder
- panic and panic disorder
- agoraphobia with and without panic disorder
- generalized anxiety states.

This book is about phobias and panic. As noted in the Introduction, I have decided to discuss them together because of the considerable overlap between these conditions and the fact that for most people, their panic and phobia are inseparable. Most people with phobias report panic attacks at some time, while most people who have panic attacks over a long period report some degree of avoidance or phobic behaviour.

I must mention three other conditions:

- post-traumatic stress disorder (PTSD)
- obsessive–compulsive disorder (OCD)
- body dysmorphic disorder.

People with these often have phobias and panic attacks that need to be treated in their own right.

Those with PTSD often experience severe anxiety relating to many situations, which may be linked to the event that triggered their condition. Thus, for example, people who have been involved in road traffic accidents and who have developed PTSD will most likely have great difficulty travelling in cars, whether as a driver or passenger. Many will find it somewhat easier to drive themselves as they fear not being in control. Sometimes, the fear of travelling in cars spreads to all situations involving public transport and, in extreme cases, they can become confined to their own homes. Sometimes simply walking along the street causes great fear and the sound of police or ambulance sirens can trigger memories of the original traumatic event.

This book may be helpful to some of you with PTSD, but I need to emphasize that, because of the wide range of other symptoms associated with this condition, a variety of treatment approaches are often necessary. In the References section at the end of this book I have included an excellent book by Dr Claudia Herbert that may be used as a comprehensive self-help guide for PTSD.

Likewise, people with OCD often have specific phobias that may be central to their condition. People with OCD commonly have phobias of dirt, germs or contamination. As with PTSD, I hope that people with OCD will find Dr Herbert's book useful. Also, see the References section for details of an excellent self-help book by Dr David Veale and Rob Willson. The Useful contacts section (p. 106) gives details of the charity OCD Action, which provides considerable help and support for people with this condition. I have personal knowledge of the charity's good work as I am its patron and have been involved in its activities over a number of years.

Body dysmorphic disorder is characterized by a preoccupation with one's appearance and often with specific parts of the body. The condition leads to phobic anxiety and avoidance, in so far as various situations, including social events, shopping and working environments, become the source of fear and distress because of the person's preoccupation with those parts of the body. More about this on p. 38.

Finally, children can have very real fears and phobias of various kinds.

To return to the various categories of anxiety states listed at the beginning, I will now say something about each of them, followed by further information on the other conditions mentioned above and children's anxieties.

Simple (specific) phobias

A phobia may be defined as a marked or persistent fear that is excessive, unreasonable or out of proportion to the danger that the situation or object presents.

There is usually a considerable amount of anticipation when someone with a phobia is aware of potential contact with a feared object or situation. Once that object or situation has been removed, however, or the person 'escapes' it, the anxiety levels return to normal.

Although the causes of phobias are not fully understood it seems very clear that avoidance of and/or repetitive escape from the object or situation makes the fear (phobia) worse. In the vast majority of cases, the person is aware that the fear associated with the phobia is excessive and/or unreasonable and may well admit to feeling silly or embarrassed about admitting the problem. Virtually every object or situation you can think of can become the object of a phobia.

The excessive fear that accompanies a phobia comprises both physical and psychological elements. Those elements form two of the central themes of this book. In the descriptions of phobias and panic that follow you will see that the fear (physical and psychological) accompanying a phobia seeps into every corner of our being. Indeed, the anticipation of the fear becomes a 'fear of fear' – often a greater problem than actually confronting the phobic object.

Simple phobias often start in early childhood and many of the people I see tell me, 'I have had this fear for as long as I can remember.' Usually there is no clear reason for the phobias to have developed, but sometimes they start after a specific traumatic event.

A lady in her thirties developed a very strong fear of bees after seeing a programme on television. Prior to this, she had no fears whatsoever, but, over a relatively short period of time following the programme, she started to go to extraordinary lengths to avoid going anywhere she thought bees might be. That included her own garden, which she had lovingly tended for several years.

This story has a happy ending, though. She was persuaded to meet a beekeeper and, having donned full beekeeping kit and after several hours of 'safe' exposure, she was still not exactly able to love and cherish bees, but did develop an interest in a very captivating topic. With the beekeeper's help (rather than a therapist's) she was able to once more enter situations where bees might be present.

The phrase 'simple phobia' does not necessarily imply that all simple phobias are mild. As with the bee phobia, some simple phobias can cause high levels of fear, extreme stress and tremendous handicaps in terms of being able to carry out the activities of daily living.

As with any anxiety disorder, or indeed any other mental health problem, phobias can be experienced at various levels of severity. In the case of simple phobias, where the anxiety is confined to a specific place, object or situation, the phobic object may rarely be encountered. I recall several years ago somebody who could not be persuaded to go on an Arctic cruise because of a phobia of icebergs. This phobia only reared its head when she was asked to go on the cruise or when she saw films or TV programmes about icebergs. After some consideration, she rejected the offer of therapy and decided that, because her phobia did not cause any disruption to her everyday life, the anxiety that might arise during treatment was not a price worth paying to overcome a phobia that rarely troubled her.

In the case of other phobias, such as the bee phobia, they may be confined to certain times of the year. At the other end of the scale, if the phobic object is essentially ever-present, the person can potentially have to face a phobia on a daily basis. Two examples of such simple phobias, which I describe further below, are a vomiting phobia and a fear of birds.

I should also say that, sometimes, simple phobias are not so simple! They may be quite complex and generate secondary behaviours, such as checking and taking additional precautions. This is particularly the case in phobias such as those of thunder and lightning or vomiting (see p. 19). Further, some simple phobias are really not simple and isolated, but are central to range of other anxiety-related problems. Also, they may be accompanied by other secondary phobias and a more general state of anxiety and panic.

This is all very interesting, but it need not concern you how phobias are classified. I mention it only because it is important to understand what the central elements of fear and avoidance are and identify all of the aspects of emotion and function that are relevant to treatment. All will become clearer later on when I explain how to develop and implement a self-help treatment plan. For now, I shall describe some of the commoner phobias or, to put it another way, those phobias that commonly come to the attention of professionals such as myself. I cannot possibly mention every phobia that exists in this book as such a list would involve, literally, thousands of objects and situations. Neither will I attempt to provide a name for each phobia. I know, for example, that the specific fear of Friday the 13th is called paraskevidekatria-phobia – this word deriving from the Greek – but you are unlikely to need to know that. In fact, I have never seen anyone who has this phobia!

There are numerous sources of lists of the names of phobias and, if you are really interested in the name for your specific phobia, I would suggest that the Internet is probably the best place to start. Having said that, in my experience, while people like to put a name to their particular problem, beyond this, what most of them want – often quite desperately – is to alleviate their fear, distress and sometimes very substantial suffering.

I hope that the descriptions of the various phobias below convey some of the principles concerning the ways in which phobias arise and encapsulate all the key features that need attention. Note that the phobias are given in no particular order of priority and nor have I attempted to provide very detailed information concerning how many people come to have such fears.

There have been several very large studies that have calculated the numbers of people with fears and phobias. The information I provide below is based on the two major studies conducted in recent years, one of which took place in the USA and one in the UK. The figures from these studies are broadly comparable and therefore constitute approximate averages.

I also need to mention a couple of issues that are relevant to people who might want to obtain more information about their phobia and discover whether it is rare or common. There are many excellent websites that provide such information. I would suggest, for very accurate statistics for the USA, you visit the National Institute for Mental Health at <www.nimh.nih.gov>. In the UK, there are several sources of very helpful and accurate information, including the Royal College of Psychiatrists at <www.rcpsych.ac.uk>. Another website that provides statistics for not only the USA and UK but also Canada and Australia is <www.cureresearch.com/statistics.htm>.

Most of the official and therefore more reliable websites use the terms 'prevalence' and 'incidence'. The *prevalence* of a phobia means the number of people who have that phobia at any one time. The word *incidence* means the annual number of people who have the condition or may also be used to mean a lifetime measure – that is, the number of people who have the condition in their lifetime. At this point it needs to be said that most phobias, apart from those which occur for a short time during childhood and then disappear, will continue to be present unless treatment is provided. The severity of a phobia, however, may wax and wane over the years.

As an indicator of how common phobias are, it is likely that 1 in 10 of the population has a phobia that would be severe enough to warrant treatment, while approximately 4 per cent of the population has a social phobia, approximately 5 per cent of the population agoraphobia or agoraphobic-like symptoms and so on. Many people participating in surveys do not reveal that they have a problem, however, so the figures from studies always have to be regarded as guides rather than exact representations of a situation.

The other thing to be said is that, although researchers do their best, after many years of reading numerous articles about the prevalence and incidence of phobias, all I can say with the utmost confidence is that these conditions are extremely common and any reasonably sized family will undoubtedly contain a number of members who have a phobia of some kind. Add to this is the fact (and by fact I mean estimate!) that approximately one in three of the population will experience a panic attack at some time during their lives and it can be seen that millions of people in the UK will have several panic attacks in any one year.

It is clear, therefore, that anxiety states, in various shapes and forms, are very common and it is worth emphasizing at the outset that they are nothing to be ashamed of. Being anxious does not mean that you lack courage or are weak. I have had the privilege, in my professional life, of meeting thousands of people with anxiety states. I have nothing but admiration for them as many have exhibited levels of courage that I could never attain and contribute so much to our community despite their fears.

Animal phobias

Earlier we encountered the story of someone with a phobia of bees, but virtually every animal could become the object of a phobia.

It is clear that there is a realistic basis, in evolutionary terms, for having a fear of many animals. A fear of animals could therefore be seen as an inbuilt and logical part of our being that has simply grown out of proportion. Surely, having a natural apprehension of animals that might kill and possibly eat you is quite reasonable.

In the UK there are, I believe, some 20,000 species of spider and none of these poses any significant risk to human beings. Thus, one might see spider phobias as being very unreasonable. If you live in Australia, however, such a fear of spiders could be considered much more reasonable, because a bite from some Australian spiders can cause very serious health problems, even death.

Likewise, while I am sure that most dog owners have nothing to fear from their particular canine friend, it is very reasonable to be wary of dogs and have some level of fear, even trying to avoid ones we don't know.

I could carry on listing the reasons for animals potentially causing harm to human beings, but, suffice it to say, a fear of them does not come out of nowhere. Many children are naturally very apprehensive of animals, but most will become more confident around them if they have some experience of them, guidance and education.

As any parent knows, the way to help a child adjust to any object or situation that causes anxiety is to demonstrate your own approach to that object or situation and then have the child approach it in graduated steps. Demonstrating a behaviour to a child is a process that psychologists call 'modelling'. Introducing a child who is afraid of dogs in such graduated steps to a friendly, docile dog and then continuing to proceed in small steps usually cures the child of that anxiety. This process is rather grandly called 'graduated exposure and habituation' – 'habituation' simply meaning getting used to something.

The commonest phobias (in the UK at least) are probably of spiders and snakes, but they are not usually severe. Most animal phobias only become apparent when the person is actually faced with that animal. In some of the cases that I see, however, people will be preoccupied with a particular animal and engage in a range of additional behaviours over and above simply avoiding the animal when they come into contact with them. Thus, I have seen people who will avoid going into certain rooms in their houses because they have, in the past, seen a spider there. In several extreme cases, I have come across people who have actually locked or boarded up sections of their houses because of their spider phobia. One man not only had no-go areas in his house but was also thrown into states of extreme panic when confronted with pictures or images of spiders on the TV and, on several occasions, had to abort shopping trips because he came across children wearing Spiderman T-shirts. In every other respect, however, this man – who eventually overcame his phobia – was a very well-adjusted and normal human being.

Some people with animal phobias become concerned about 'contamination' – that surfaces have been contaminated by an animal. They may then involve themselves in secondary behaviours, such as extensive cleaning rituals. Such behaviour is an example of when a phobia is actually part of another anxiety disorder – in this case, an obsessive–compulsive disorder. Then, there is usually evidence that the person had some inclination to obsessions and compulsions anyway.

Returning to the vast majority of people with animal phobias, these usually lend themselves to treatment by simple, graduated exposure, which I describe in more detail in Chapter 7. For the moment, suffice it to say that treatment involving a very gradual approach to the phobic object and learning to become more confident and less anxious around it can often achieve a cure. Most research studies of animal phobias report success rates of 90 per cent or more people cured or at least very much improved.

Flying phobia

Fear of flying is very common. Indeed, some surveys have suggested that up to 40 per cent of people experience some anxiety while flying.

Many people manage their fears by simply gritting their teeth and concluding their flight saying, 'I'm so pleased that's over!' Others take modest amounts of alcohol or follow the advice given on various airlines' websites suggesting that doctors can prescribe mild tranquillizers. Indeed, the very judicious use of mild tranquillizing drugs for people who fly perhaps only once or twice a year and whose levels of anxiety are mild to moderate is, in my opinion, quite reasonable.

The use of alcohol may be a problem because, instead of having one drink and waiting for that to take effect, the person may consume a large quantity of alcohol in a short space of time and become intoxicated. This may even lead to the person either becoming so incapacitated that he or she is not allowed to board the flight or else engaging in unwelcome disruptive behaviour.

One other problem that I frequently encounter is when people mix a prescription drug – usually something in the Valium family – with alcohol. The combination of such substances may lead to unwelcome levels of intoxication.

Flying phobias may be divided into two categories. First, there are people who fear flying because they are scared of the aircraft crashing. Second, there are those who fear flying because they are in a confined space with no opportunity to escape. Sometimes people have a combination of these fears.

Fears of the aircraft crashing are, in my opinion, generally easier to deal with than fears of being confined. Information and education about aircraft and flying in general may often lead to a substantial reduction in anxiety. Thus, it is essential that people are taught about matters that often trigger anxiety, such as the noises accompanying wing flap changes or the undercarriage. Turbulence often causes considerable fear, so explaining how aircraft are built to withstand the stresses and strains that occur during this phenomenon can help. These factors are often more important in assisting people than simply giving them the statistics that, considering the vast number of flights taking place every day, the number of crashes is comparatively small. If you are in an aeroplane that is bumping and juddering and you become fixated on the safety instructions (including references to safety positions and the whistle for attracting attention), such numbers are cold comfort!

For people who fear being enclosed in an aircraft without any means of escape, this may be linked with other fears of enclosed situations, such as lifts, underground trains and tunnels. In many instances, however, there is no such link.

It is interesting to note that several people I have seen have been able to travel in small aircraft, which have a much poorer safety record than jumbo jets. That is because, in a small aircraft, flying with a pilot they know personally, they always have the option of asking the pilot to land at the nearest airfield. Thus, they perceive that they are more in control of the situation than they would be in a jumbo jet.

When I ask people with such fears why the enclosed space without a means of escape is a problem, they will often reply along the lines of, 'I have a fear of losing control.' Probing this fear even further, the person often reveals that losing control may mean a number of things, from going mad to becoming crazy in their behaviour, to becoming incontinent, vomiting and so on. Thus, sometimes a specific fear, such as that of vomiting, is linked with a fear of vomiting in other situations. More often than not, however, the core fear – fear of flying – is confined to flying situations. Interestingly, most people with a flying phobia do not have a fear of heights.

For many people, the commonsense approach to flying is to be greatly commended – that is, if you are afraid of flying, fly more often and, the more you do it, the easier it will become. This does not necessarily hold true for everyone, though, and there is, in fact, well-documented research literature on anxiety among flight crew. It is worth saying here that such anxiety states are taken very seriously by airlines and the health screening for pilots is, in the UK at least (and probably in the rest of the Western world), exemplary.

Flying phobias are recognized as being so common that most of the larger airlines offer courses to help people overcome them. These usually comprise an introduction, with presentations given by pilots, who provide the necessary knowledge about how aircraft fly, the technical side of aviation and the training of pilots. This is followed by a discussion with fellow flying phobics and the support that comes from knowing that you are not alone. During this discussion, the pilots are present to answer any further questions.

The next part usually consists of a talk by a psychologist about the psychological aspects of phobias, how fear operates and what to do when you become anxious. The psychologist will demonstrate how relaxation and breathing exercises can diminish your physical fear and describe other strategies that you can use to reduce anxiety and panic.

The day ends with a flight on an aircraft accompanied by the psychologist and pilots. During the flight, the pilots provide a running commentary from the flight deck on the various phases of the flight.

Generally speaking, even quite severe phobics benefit from such courses. One of the more powerful aspects is meeting others with similar fears, who all help each other to overcome the central phobia. Although I can do a great deal to help someone referred to me for individual treatment, in the majority of cases I advise people to attend one of these courses as, in my opinion, this provides one of the most effective ways of dealing with the problem.

One final thing to note about flying phobias is that they are, perhaps, the best example of fears that are strengthened by anticipation. Very often the anticipation of the forthcoming flight takes place over a period of months and the anticipatory anxiety leads to the person's level of arousal becoming more and more heightened and, in many respects, anticipation strengthens the fear. Indeed, anticipation is a key feature of many phobias. The social phobic will anticipate the dinner party, the person with fears of underground travel may anticipate his journey to work and so on. For the once-a-year flyer who is undertaking the flight because of a much wished for holiday, however, the anticipation forms a very important component of the whole fear process and may, indeed, lead to many months of life being dominated by anxiety. It is, therefore, often very important to deal with this anticipation as a problem in its own right.

There are many things you can do to help break the pattern of anticipation. I often ask clients to drive to the local airport and invest in parking at the short-term car park so that they can visit the airport terminal and simply get used to the atmosphere of an airport. Many airports offer vantage points so that you can actually see aircraft taking off and landing. This is very often a useful exercise.

There are also other ways of preparing oneself for a flight. Some computer games offer flight simulations and, for many years, I have also asked people to listen to sound effects such as interior aircraft noises, engine sounds and so on, as this exposure serves to reduce fear.

There are different motivations for seeking treatment for a flying phobia. Some people simply want to be able to travel once or twice a year to go on holiday. For an increasing number of people, however, flying can be required for their work, either occasionally or even daily. It is surprising how common it is to hear of people who fly from home to London and back every week, commuting from Scotland or Northern Ireland, for example, or working in London from Tuesday morning to Thursday evening. In addition, with access to frequent flights from numerous airports across the UK, there are now many people who fly to parts of Europe and back on the same day for a meeting or else to go away for the weekend.

If people wish to fly only once a year or perhaps less often, the gains that are to be had from treatment, whether this be self-help, professional or one of the airlines' courses, may be short-lived. I always stress to those I meet who are thinking about treatment that, in order for gains to be continued and maintained, they need to then make regular flights. I am pleased to say that at least three of the people I have worked with have graduated from being flying phobics to enjoying passenger travel, then went on to learn to fly themselves, obtaining private pilots' licences. One of them not only has a licence to fly aeroplanes but he also flies helicopters, hang-gliders and gliders – a true case of conquering his fears!

Heights phobias

The fear of heights is quite common and many people would not even call it a phobia, although technically it is. Thus, when talking about the London Eye, for example, it is common to hear people say, 'You wouldn't catch me going up there!' The same thing occurs with the Monument, the Whispering Gallery in St Paul's Cathedral and the Empire State Building.

As with other specific phobias, height phobias may be connected to other fears or anxieties. The nature of the phobia is often quite different from one person to another. Some people manage to be in very high places and feel perfectly calm, providing there is something, even if it is glass, between themselves and the drop to earth. I know several people who have been to the top of the CN Tower in Toronto and have been able to stand in the middle on the glass floor and look down to the earth below without any difficulty. Yet, these same people have a real problem with leaning over a balcony in a theatre or the atrium of a shop.

Some people have great trouble with all heights, whether or not there is an exterior wall of glass. One person who came to me had resigned from her job in the City of London when she was relocated to a high-rise building with glass-fronted offices. Many people report that being on the edge of any precipice makes them feel that they are going to be drawn over it. It seems that some people have developed an abnormally sensitive balance system (called the vestibular system, which is in the inner ear). It is certainly true that, as the vestibular system of the ear deteriorates with age, a fear of heights may become more intense.

Sometimes a fear of heights is accompanied by a fear of looking up at tall buildings as the person feels very dizzy and uncomfortable. If this happens in an area with many skyscrapers, it may be a manifestation of a fear of enclosed spaces. Equally, however, it may simply be that looking up and craning one's head and neck back triggers the body's receptors in the neck and ear to react.

People come for treatment for their height phobia for a variety of reasons. For example, one young man attended because his work necessitated him travelling across the Queen Elizabeth II Bridge, which forms part of the Dartford Crossing. This huge, four-lane suspension bridge is very high up for quite a long way as it spans the Thames and extends some distance either side. He is not alone. Indeed, panic attacks among people who travel across this bridge are so common that, for many years, the owners of the bridge offered a service wherein people with such anxieties could be accompanied by a staff member. At the time of writing, this service has been withdrawn, not because of lack of demand but because of its funding and logistical implications.

> A young woman, a teacher, came to see me because, as she said, she had 'run out of excuses' as to why she could not go on the school ski trip. When she started her job, she had volunteered the information to the school that, as a child, she had learned to ski to a good standard. What she did not go on to say, however, was that, in her late teenage years, she became increasingly concerned that she might topple from the ski lift. On one occasion she said that she was frozen with fear and panic and after that holiday experience she determined never to go skiing again. Because of the pressure from her employers, though, she sought treatment with me and, eventually, managed to conquer her fear. It is worth noting that at no time was she afraid of the views from the top of the mountain and, in fact, was very pleased to conquer her phobia because the skiing itself was something she really enjoyed.

I have seen several people who have declined going on cruises because large modern cruise ships often have a very large atrium in the middle, sometimes up to 15 storeys high. In such cases, the motivation for treatment often comes not from individuals themselves but from their spouses or friends and relatives. In this respect, treatment is sometimes hampered by a lack of motivation on the part of the individuals themselves.

This highlights an important aspect of treatment. If you set about conquering a fear for others rather than for yourself, you may become resentful that you are being put under pressure to do something that causes you distress with no apparent benefit to you. While some people who are 'doing it for others' complete treatment successfully, others give up shortly after their first appointment or when they are first confronted with a treatment situation that causes the anxiety.

A fear of high places may be accompanied by a fear of any situation where there is an edge. The commonest example of such an edge is a train or underground platform. In these cases, people worry about being drawn to the edge and falling or jumping off it against their will, straight into the path of an oncoming train.

Over the years I have seen literally hundreds of people with height phobias and I have to say that there is no standard form such phobias take. As with other phobias, each person has his or her own story and some of the features of that story seem somewhat contradictory, as we saw with the teacher who loved skiing but hated ski lifts. In each case, despite such apparent contradictions, if you listen to the person carefully enough and ask the right questions, there is an internal consistency that is not immediately obvious.

Weather phobias

Over the years I have seen a number of people with weather phobias. The majority of these are phobias of thunder and lightning, but others fear snow or heavy rain.

Weather phobias are generally linked to a fear of physical injury or death. Thus, a fear of rain is usually linked to a fear of flooding and drowning, while a fear of lightning is really a fear of being struck by it and thus electrocuted. Occasionally, however, people who fear thunder actually have a phobia of loud noises.

Most weather phobics indulge in checking and protective behaviours of one kind or another. Some obsessively check weather forecasts and may even ring the Meteorological Office to discuss the weather with a member of staff there. Checking may also include them taking their own detailed barometric readings and obsessively watching the sky. One person who did this sort of thing told me that he also rang friends and relatives at frequent intervals to ask them, 'What's the weather like in your part of the world?' This was usually followed by the question, 'Do you think we'll have a storm tonight?' In several cases I have seen people with storm phobias who have created a 'safe room', like those found in areas prone to tornados and hurricanes. I think nearly everyone would agree that having a soundproof room, with a reinforced door and a safe in the floor for valuables, is an extraordinary level of protection for someone who lives in a leafy suburb of London. Nevertheless, I have seen more than one case of such measures being taken. That some people go to such lengths demonstrates that phobias can be severe, although the majority of people with weather phobias would not go to such extremes.

Fear of dentists

Dental phobias are very common. This can lead to years of avoiding going to the dentist, which, in turn can cause a wide range of problems, from the cosmetic to the downright painful.

Fortunately, students at schools of dentistry are now provided with a great deal of information concerning dental phobias and treatment. Indeed, I was recently pleased to hear from the young dentist who came to me for treatment (for another condition – not a fear of dentists) that she had attended a number of courses regarding the management of anxious patients. She told me that she obtained a great deal of satisfaction from treating patients who had had dental phobias for many years and, for that reason, had failed to receive the dental treatment they needed.

Professor Isaac Marks, who was my original teacher in the field of fears and phobias, had his very comprehensive book on phobias – *Fears, Phobias and Rituals* – published in 1987. In it he tells the story of how Queen Elizabeth I was 'excessively tormented' by pain caused by a decaying tooth, but would not have it extracted because of the pain that would accompany the procedure. He tells of how she was eventually persuaded to undergo treatment by the Bishop of London. The bishop – an old man with not many teeth to spare – underwent the extraction of one of his teeth in the presence of Queen Elizabeth and this encouraged her to submit to the operation herself.

Things have improved a lot since Elizabethan times, but people still fear dentists for a range of reasons. Sometimes it is a worry about being confined in the dentist's chair, without ready means of escape. Sometimes it is the fear of having a panic attack and being humiliated in front of the dentist. Sometimes it is a fear of having a procedure that will cause pain. Others fear that their airways will be blocked and they won't be able to breathe. People also experience combinations of two or more or even all of these factors and, indeed, other fears.

As noted above, dental phobias may lead to considerable avoidance behaviour and, sadly, many people suffer years of tooth decay and infection before finally succumbing to seeing a dentist. I have not yet mentioned the fear of injections, because injection phobias themselves, although they may form part of dental phobias, form a group of phobias in their own right (see p. 21).

The manifestations of dental phobias are wide ranging. Sometimes only the person concerned knows that he or she is afraid and keeps that fear hidden. Often, however, the physical manifestations of anxiety will be obvious. For example, the person may become very tense or sweat profusely. Another symptom is an increase in the 'gag reflex'. This is a normal reflex that involves the muscles of the mouth and pallet rejecting any object put into the mouth and then a spasm of the mouth and retching, but the person's nervousness can lead to hypersensitivity so that this reflex occurs much more readily than is normal.

What often helps is for the dentist to say, 'If at any time you want me to stop, just signal.' In some cases, just telling the dentist that you are anxious will help. Disclosing rather than hiding the fear is often a relief in itself.

Dentists use a variety of methods to assist the anxious person. A graduated approach is always useful and, especially with anxious children, it is important for patients to feel that they are involved in the dental procedure. For example, it is useful to allow them to familiarize themselves with all the equipment and what they are used for. Sometimes the suction devices used to extract saliva from the mouth may cause anxiety and adjusting the level of suction is sometimes important. My own dentist uses a camera to show people a view of their mouths that they normally never see and tells me that this can be very effective in helping people with anxiety.

When people consult me for treatment of a dental phobia, I always say that the first step is to involve the dentist who will eventually see them. In the case of those who have not seen a dentist for many years, I have a list of dentists in my own area I know are very skilled at handling anxious patients. In severe cases, it is important to begin by simply exposing the person to the smells of the dental surgery and the equipment used. Many people have told me that the smell of the dental surgery alone is enough to trigger a panic attack.

The main problem, once again, is anticipation. This may be the anticipation of severe pain or simply 'being trapped'. Modern dentistry involves much less pain than in the past and, although some dental procedures are a little painful, that pain is managed to minimize it and any there is is usually short-lived. Those who are really anxious all the same may benefit from practising relaxation techniques or, as a last resort, taking a short-acting tranquillizer. Some dentists learn such techniques during their training or subsequently.

Overall, dental phobias usually respond well to treatment. I think this is partly because having healthy teeth that look good is reinforcement in itself and people have a great determination to face their fears.

Interestingly, some dentists have a fear of carrying out dental procedures. In some cases this involves a concern about the patient seeing that they are anxious. In one case the dentist had a mild tremor that resulted from being under stress. Although this only appeared occasionally and did not in any way affect his work, he became preoccupied that the tremor would appear during a procedure (this had never happened) and the patient would notice. The problem was compounded by his anticipating that this would happen, which strengthened his fear.

In another case, a dentist developed a fear that she might blush (another very common fear) and, despite using large amounts of make-up to conceal any blushing, she eventually found herself unable to work because of the extent of her fear. She is, unfortunately, not alone as several dentists seen by myself and colleagues restrict the types of work that they do because of such fears. In some of the more serious cases, as with my dentist with the blushing worry, they stop working as dentists altogether.

I am of the opinion that dental surgery is one of the most demanding of the healthcare professions. Dentists spend much of each day in close proximity to patients, much closer than most GPs. In addition, they maybe 'catch' the anxiety of many of their patients. This 'infectivity of anxiety' is a phenomenon that is well known. Any therapist who spends a great deal of time in the presence of people demonstrating high levels of anxiety will tell you that it certainly rubs off. Many years ago I was involved in the treatment of people who had very severe levels of agoraphobia. As part of their treatment, I would accompany them to shopping centres and similar locations to expose them in a group to situations that they feared and previously avoided. They were often very tense in the anticipatory period and we often spent three or more hours in the phobic situation until their fears reduced. I can certainly testify, first-hand, that one by-product of these treatment sessions was the need for me to go home and unwind because afterwards I myself felt very tense and uptight. I know that this experience is shared by many of my colleagues.

Incidentally, this method of treatment is now used much less than it was. This is for two central reasons. The first is that helping people to help themselves seems, for the majority, to be the best approach and such exposure can be equally successfully carried out using a family member as a cotherapist. The other reason is simply resources. I was fortunate to be trained in an era when the demands on treatment resources were much less and it was possible to give people many hours of therapist-aided exposure to their fears. Over the years, however, although there has been a growth in the number of therapists in the NHS, the demand for treatment has grown a lot more so therapists simply do not have the time to devote to such sessions.

Vomiting phobias

Vomiting phobias are one of the commonest phobias that I see in my clinical work and vary quite considerably in terms of their severity. They generally take one of two forms, but sometimes a combination of the two.

The first form is a phobia of seeing other people vomit. The second is the fear of them vomiting themselves. The first form is, in many ways, a much easier phobia to treat. The second may cause a wide range of avoidance and checking behaviours, as well as generally being preoccupied with thoughts about it.

Many people with vomiting phobias adapt their eating habits to avoid certain foodstuffs that they associate with being sick. So, for example, they may avoid mayonnaise and shellfish and, when eating out, foods known to 'upset the tummy', such as curries, spicy foods and anything that they remotely connect with food poisoning.

It is also very common to see people with this phobia become obsessed with sell-by dates and discard perfectly good foods because of fears of contamination. One client I saw found a yogurt pot in her fridge that was one day out of date. She became so preoccupied with thoughts about it being out of date that she emptied the entire fridge and adjoining freezer because she thought that the yogurt might have contaminated the remaining food in the fridge and freezer.

A vomiting phobia may lead to other preoccupations, too. I have come across many people who have become concerned about their children's health and the possibility that their children may have been infected with a tummy bug by other children at school. Unfortunately, this may lead to serious problems. In several cases that I have seen, parents have withdrawn their children from school because of this fear. The problem with fears of contamination, which underpin vomiting, is that they may lead to behaviour that could certainly be described as obsessive and checking and cleaning rituals may also result. The advent of antibacterial gels has led to a marked increase in the number of people with vomiting phobia. They will use these gels and a variety of wet wipes and tissues to ensure that they are not contaminated.

One common reason for women being referred for treatment is a fear of vomiting in pregnancy. Sadly, I have seen several cases of women who have avoided becoming pregnant, although they would dearly love to have children, because of the fear that they may vomit while they are pregnant. In fact, for those who do become pregnant and have morning sickness, this often cures their problem.

Vomiting phobias may also lead to an avoidance of alcohol. This may be linked to not only a fear that the alcohol may produce nausea and vomiting but also of it being essentially a mind-altering drug, leading to some form of loss of control.

Vomiting phobias are categorized as simple phobias, but clients who come to see me often require quite extensive treatment over several weeks or months. That is because it is necessary to approach the problems gradually and there are so many different aspects to them, not least of which are all the secondary behaviours that arise. Although some respond to a rapid approach, many people need to abandon their checking rituals and safety behaviours, such as the use of antibacterial gels and wipes, very gradually. This is quite a challenge for therapists as they need to balance helping their clients to advance as much as possible with ensuring that they do not feel the treatment tasks they are given are unmanageable. Treatment may involve exposing the client to video clips of vomiting, imagining him- or herself vomiting and eating previously avoided foods. Treatment varies, however, as each person is unique and, for it to be effective, it needs to be carefully thought through.

Incontinence phobias and irritable bowel syndrome

Irritable bowel syndrome (IBS) is often experienced by people who have phobias and panic attacks and is often unresponsive to treatment. IBS can, in turn, lead to a phobia of incontinence and may complicate other phobias, such as a vomiting phobia.

IBS is an umbrella term for a number of different conditions. These conditions have several characteristics in common and it is true to say that most forms of IBS comprise both physiological and psychological components.

IBS is extremely common, some textbooks stating that about 50 per cent of people who are referred to gastroenterologists are referred for this condition.

The main symptoms are usually abdominal pain, altered bowel habits and constipation alternating with diarrhoea. The pain may be of a dull or aching variety, but sometimes can be knife-like. The location of the pain can also move so that sometimes it is in the lower left or right side of the abdomen, while at other times it will be higher up in the middle of the abdomen, just under the ribs.

Sometimes the stools are very frequent and watery, particularly in the morning. This frequency of bowel activity in the morning often means people avoid going out before it slows down or ceases. This may develop into a more general avoidance of situations where toilets are not readily accessible and gradually into a severe general phobia of going anywhere where one is not close by.

Sometimes people take regular amounts of antidiarrhoea medications, which may make constipation more severe. Yet others become so worried about the diarrhoea that they restrict their intake of all foods that they believe (often incorrectly) cause it, often having what is, in effect, a diet very low in fibre. This, of course, is generally unhealthy and may cause further problems.

All these aspects mean that IBS causes considerable anxiety and leads to all kinds of avoidance behaviour. Some people with IBS are just generally anxious, some have symptoms of OCD and others have no apparent anxiety or, indeed, any other mental health problems.

This is a condition that appears to have several causes and, as far as anxiety is concerned, it has something of a chicken and egg dimension to it. It is normal to become anxious that you might suddenly need to find a toilet, but, at the same time, that anxiety could cause an increase in bowel activity. Similarly, IBS may lead to nausea, which, in turn, may lead to the worsening of a vomiting phobia. Thus, the causation of IBS is something that remains the source of debate and controversy.

From the physiological point of view, it seems clear that some people have particularly sensitive intestinal tracts and their muscle activity is greater than normal. From the perspective of treatment, it may be greatly improved by targeting any phobic behaviour. Whatever the situation, IBS remains prevalent and, generally speaking, needs medical as well as psychological interventions to bring it under control. Having said that, it is clear that, for most people with IBS, there is no absolute cure for this condition and, mysteriously, it tends to wax and wane over a lifetime.

Blood, injury and injection phobias

These phobias are very common. Most of us will know someone who faints at the sight of blood or while having an injection. The proper medical term for this is vascovagal syncope, for those of you who like to know these things!

Nearly half of young children have a mild fear of blood and this is more common in females than males. That there is a general underlying predisposition to feeling queasy at the sight of blood is very obvious when new medical students attend their first anatomy class and are confronted with a dead body that they soon have to dissect! The vast majority of them learn how to control this natural reaction quite quickly and, during their training, soon get used to blood, injuries, injections and so on. It is interesting that some doctors, however, still feel some queasiness on being confronted with blood and injury, which may explain why they practise in branches of medicine where they never come across them. It is only as a result of my years of treating doctors for various problems that I know this to be true as the doctors themselves are unlikely to admit it to their colleagues or disclose their fears in surveys.

If someone with a blood, injury and injection fear faints, this is unusual because, in the vast majority of people with phobias, the heart rate increases and blood pressure rises on encountering the feared object and blood pressure needs to fall for a person to faint. Thus, although people with phobias often report feeling faint, they are very seldom – if ever – in danger of actually fainting because their blood pressure is increased rather than decreased, so the feelings of faintness are connected instead with physiological symptoms of arousal.

During periods of low blood pressure, for reasons of gravity, the blood supply to the brain is decreased. Fainting is the body's response to low blood pressure as, simply, if you fall over in a faint, being horizontal restores the blood supply to your brain. We have known for many years that people who faint at the sight of blood or during injections or blood taking do so because their heart rate reduces and their blood pressure falls. Indeed, in many cases, the heart actually stops beating for several seconds. Although this might sound very dramatic, the act of fainting restores – after a period of some recovery – normal cardiac function. The reduction in heart and blood pressure is, in itself, harmless, even in people with significant cardiovascular disease. In some cases, the blood pressure and pulse fall, but actual fainting does not occur because the blood pressure remains at a level that means some blood is going to the brain. In such cases, the person complains of feeling dizzy and very often sick. Following the faint there may be some twitching of muscles, but there is rarely any other problem.

While the treatment for this group of phobias, like any other phobia, involves gradually increasing exposure to the cause of the phobia, therapists need to also take into account the physiological characteristics that accompany them. For example, it is useful to learn techniques to raise blood pressure.

One tried and tested method is to tense the upper body while holding your breath. If people carry out the tensing procedure while, at the same time, seeing their blood pressure rise and fall by using one of the commonly available electronic blood pressure measuring machines and watching the digital displays of measurements, they can see clearly how their body reacts to what they are doing. Sometimes, just understanding the physiology of the phobia in this way is beneficial – knowledge really is power!

The gradual exposure of the person to the feared object or situation can be done in a number of ways. In the case of an injection phobia, for example, I often ask people to begin by handling syringes and needles. When they grow comfortable doing this, then they can progress to using sterile needles to break the surface of the skin and, eventually, to having blood taken or being given an injection of sterile water.

It is generally advisable for people lie down during the initial stages of treatment, to assist gravity, as we have seen, and ensure that blood gets to the brain, overcoming any feelings of faintness. It also helps if they can observe others having their blood taken and I quite commonly ask people to watch video clips of such situations. Again, many people find it helpful to lie down while watching these clips, to reduce any feelings of dizziness. Similarly, I have asked one of my colleagues to take some blood from my arm while my client looks on from the comfort of a sofa.

In this way, very gradually, people find that they can become desensitized to injections and able to have blood taken or injections given in a sitting or standing position. Alternatively, people can warn their doctor or a nurse who is taking blood or giving them an injection of their phobia and opt to lie down while these procedures are carried out.

I have seen and treated several people with such phobias who have required chemotherapy. I am pleased to report that when they persisted with the treatment I have described, the outcomes have usually been excellent. One person, without any prompting from me I have to say, thought that his treatment might be assisted by exposing himself to blood and injury and so he went to a boxing dinner where there were to be four bouts. Unfortunately for him, but perhaps fortunately for the boxers, none of the fights involved any blood letting so he came away disappointed. Nevertheless, the very fact that he could go where he might encounter blood greatly boosted his confidence.

From the research evidence available it can be concluded that these phobias are most probably genetically determined and, rather than being seen as a psychological problem, we should see them as a physical problem with psychological consequences.

Illness phobias

Illness phobias are sometimes categorized as simple phobias and, indeed, sometimes that is exactly what they are – simple, isolated fears. More often, however, illness phobias are part of a more wide-ranging pattern of anxiety, so they are now more commonly referred to as health anxiety.

Illness phobias are also referred to as hypochondriasis. The term 'hypochondriac' derives from this term, but tends to be used in a rather derogatory way so is generally not used by health professionals.

Whatever you call the condition, though, illness phobias are often very disabling and have consequences for others, in so far as they often affect other family members and society as a whole. On the latter point, people with health anxiety often consume huge amounts of healthcare resources (I must emphasize that this is through no fault of their own), which costs a great deal per year.

In some ways, positive developments in medicine and dissemination of information via the Internet have caused the problem to become more pronounced. It seems clear to me that the advent of whole body scanning, a facility offered by several private companies, may result in an even greater preoccupation with health and, quite often, cause unnecessary anxiety.

A 45-year-old woman was reassured by her doctor that she was in excellent health, but decided to have what she called 'a total MOT'. The MOT consisted of a scan of her whole body and revealed a small shadow on her brain. This led to her being referred to a neurologist and undergoing tests to discover whether or not she had a brain tumour.

After literally weeks of waiting, the woman was in a state of extreme anxiety and even went so far as to make provisions for her untimely demise. Eventually, the cause of the shadow was identified as a small area of calcification that may have dated back to a childhood head injury. It was absolutely harmless.

A man who had previously been pronounced very fit and was accomplished in extreme sports (extreme sports involve pushing your body to the limit by climbing and descending mountains rapidly, jumping out of helicopters on to ski slopes and the like) decided to ignore his GP's opinion and go to one of the health insurance companies offering health screening. While he underwent exercise testing (his heart's functioning was measured to produce an electrocardiogram while he was exercising), he was found to have some abnormal wave patterns.

This led to no fewer than six different, complex investigations being carried out and the man naturally experienced a great deal of anxiety. In subsequent examinations by the cardiologist he saw, he exhibited high blood pressure. In the event, these high blood pressure readings turned out to be a manifestation of his anxiety (white coat hypertension – see p. 26), rather than the result of a true problem. When he eventually saw a cardiologist who had an interest in sportspeople, his abnormal wave form was identified as being simply a manifestation of his exceptional cardiac fitness. These unnecessary investigations led to this man coming to see me for treatment for panic attacks. Fortunately, he responded to cognitive behaviour therapy fairly quickly and the last time I heard from him was when he sent me a Christmas card telling me about his latest feat in the Himalayas.

Health anxieties tend to change with the times. Twenty years ago AIDS phobias were extremely common and numerous people came to professionals like myself with a preoccupation that they may have contracted AIDS by shaking hands with an infected person, sitting on a red spot on a seat on the underground or meeting a homosexual person at a dinner party. Since then, people have generally become much more informed about AIDS and HIV infection. Now, HIV infection, if properly managed, in most cases does not develop into anything more serious. As a result of these developments, the number of people with AIDS phobias has somewhat diminished. Nevertheless, testing for HIV is now a major industry and, unfortunately, some people needlessly have HIV tests very frequently. In these cases, repeated testing often leads to an increase, rather than a decrease, in anxiety and is not to be recommended unless a person's lifestyle and so on mean that it is a sensible precaution.

During my professional career, I have seen peaks and troughs in the frequency of various illnesses and them being the focus of people's worries. At the time of writing, swine flu is the greatest source of anxiety and some people have very quickly developed fully fledged phobias of the condition despite it being only a few months since it was first recognized.

Creutzfeldt-Jakob disease, more commonly known as mad cow disease, was another condition that caused considerable anxiety and I recall many people avoiding roast dinners and hamburgers. The perennial favourites, however, remain heart disease, cancer, Alzheimer's disease and multiple sclerosis.

The way in which the focus on various diseases alters is an interesting, but possibly not such a significant part of the condition. The best way to view health anxiety is to see it as a condition that simply happens to focus on a particular disease at a particular time and is a part of a person's underlying predisposition to worry about his or her health.

Some people develop health anxiety following a traumatic event. Examples include people who have suffered a heart attack and recovered, but who are affected by their brush with death. They often develop such levels of avoidance that they abstain from all types of exercise and thus, ironically, increase their risk of further cardiac problems rather than reduce it.

I have also seen several cases of health anxiety that seem to have been triggered by reactions to medical procedures, such as epidural injections. In these instances the medical procedures seem to have caused symptoms of increased physiological arousal, such as a pounding heart, chest pain, breathlessness and so on, that, in turn, have led to a pattern of anxiety and avoidance.

Some people develop their phobia following an extreme allergic reaction (sometimes referred to as anaphylactic shock) following a wasp sting or a reaction to a medication. In several such cases, the health phobia has developed in people who apparently had no health concerns prior to the traumatic event. In these cases, the phobia is often accompanied by behaviours that are aimed at ensuring their safety and, thus, they avoid certain situations and so on. One woman, who developed an allergic reaction to penicillin, resolutely refused to take any medicines and came to me for treatment because she had extremely high blood pressure (not caused by her anxiety) that required urgent treatment. Because of her phobia, she felt unable to take her blood pressure medication. Once more, this story had a happy ending, but she required more than 30 sessions before she was able to begin her course of antihypertensive drugs.

Although in later chapters I describe treatment approaches for phobias, it is impossible in a book such as this to convey information about all the possible treatments. I will, however, say this: successful treatment for health phobias should (and in my opinion must) involve your GP. Your GP is at the centre of your healthcare. I say this particularly because people with health anxieties or illness phobias often visit their GPs frequently without telling them about the true nature of their fears. GPs, because of the pressure on their time, will frequently not therefore obtain the true picture of what is going on so will not be able to advise them appropriately. In my experience, however, the vast majority of GPs, once they know that there is a problem with health anxiety, turn out to be great allies.

White coat hypertension (blood pressure phobias)

One problem I see regularly is people who are anxious diagnosed as having high blood pressure. Quite often, they will say that just going to see the doctor or nurse to have their blood pressure taken makes them feel very anxious. There is then a concern about whether or not the blood pressure readings are reliable. Of course some of them may truly have high blood pressure, which needs treatment, but some of them do not.

First, some information about blood pressure. Blood pressure readings – for example 130/70, or, 130 over 70 – relate to the pressure of blood measured in millimetres of mercury, usually using the person's left arm. The readings come from the blood pressure cuff wrapped around the person's arm being inflated and deflated so that the pressure in the main artery running down the arm is recorded. This is a reliable way of estimating whether or not the pressure of the blood in the body is reasonable.

The top figure – in our example above, 130 – is the pressure of blood, in millimetres of mercury, when the heart is pumping blood out. This process is known as systole, so this is the systolic reading. The lower figure – in this case 70 – is the pressure of blood, in millimetres of mercury, when the heart is at rest. This part of the cardiac cycle is known as diastole, so this is the diastolic reading.

Over the years there has been some debate about what measurements should be deemed as normal and what measurements should be deemed as abnormal and therefore require treatment.

Of course, blood pressure can rise dramatically with exercise or strenuous physical activity. Likewise, it may rise because of anxiety, anger or other strong emotions. The very high blood pressure readings that might be recorded if you were to take a cold shower after a sauna or having sprinted 100 metres are, in general terms, of no consequence as a reasonably healthy body can deal with such stresses for short periods. Usually, our blood vessels are elastic enough to cope with temporary, even high, rises in blood pressure. Blood pressure only becomes a problem when above normal readings are sustained for the majority or all of the time.

What is normal? Ideally, blood pressure should be around 120/80. However, anything up to 140/90 is generally deemed to be acceptable. In people who may be more vulnerable to the effects of raised blood pressure, such as those with diabetes, 130/85 is a more acceptable limit. It is important to emphasize that blood pressure readings may vary considerably, so one isolated reading should not be a cause for worry. For that reason, doctors like to measure blood pressure when you are in a relatively relaxed state and take the average over a period of time. When doctors are unsure, they use a 24-hour monitoring device that records blood pressure at regular intervals during that time. This gives doctors a picture of how the individual's blood pressure varies over time and it is then possible to establish what the average reading is.

The causes of high blood pressure essentially boil down to two sets of factors. The first set is genetic. It is clear that some people, who may be otherwise fit and healthy, are simply biologically predisposed to having high blood pressure.

The second set of factors are to do with lifestyle. We know that lifestyle choices are very likely to increase blood pressure. In no particular order of importance they are:

- eating too much salt
- eating insufficient fruit and vegetables
- being overweight
- not taking sufficient exercise
- drinking too much alcohol
- smoking
- being subject to stress.

You may read this last point and automatically assume that this means if you are anxious, your blood pressure will be high. This is far from the truth. Over the years I have seen literally thousands of people with anxiety states and only a minority of them also have high blood pressure. Stress may not involve an anxiety state. It may, instead, be caused by working in an environment where there is constant pressure to meet impossible targets. Thus, although psychological factors are important in high blood pressure, the other factors listed above are probably responsible for a great many more instances of it than where there is anxiety alone.

High blood pressure is one of the major health problems of our age. It can cause problems with the heart, which may lead to stroke and kidney failure. It may also cause a range of other problems, including some types of dementia. If you have other health problems, such as high levels of cholesterol or diabetes, high blood pressure serves to compound them.

Doctors increasingly realize that, although modern drug treatments have fewer side effects than the older drugs, perhaps the most important way to help is to deal with lifestyle factors. There is plenty of research to suggest that taking adequate exercise, stopping smoking, eating a healthy diet and losing weight can make the difference between having a blood pressure problem that requires treatment and is potentially fatal and having a healthy blood pressure level, which equates with a good quality of life.

How do people with white coat hypertension or blood pressure phobia find out what their blood pressure really is? As noted above, doctors will generally want to take a number of readings on different occasions or use a 24-hour monitoring device to do this. The problem with such strategies is that people with very high levels of anxiety about having their blood pressure taken will remain anxious every time their blood pressure is taken and during the 24 hours a monitor is worn. Thus, in such individuals, their true blood pressure may never be revealed.

One answer to this problem is for people to measure their own blood pressure using the kinds of electronic devices that are available from high street pharmacies. These are calibrated to give accurate readings and your pharmacist can advise on the most accurate machine. People can then take readings periodically and try out different relaxation and breathing exercises to reduce their anxiety.

Nevertheless, use of these machines may lead to other problems. I have certainly come across a number of people who became obsessed with recording their blood pressure, so it can become a problem in its own right. This qualification aside, if home monitoring is used sensibly and, ideally, with the cooperation of your GP, it can be very helpful in determining exactly what your blood pressure is.

Returning to the lifestyle remedies for high blood pressure, you will notice that these will also reduce anxiety and, really, it makes sense to stick to these central messages: exercise regularly, eat sensibly and don't smoke.

Social phobia or social anxiety disorder

The American Psychiatric Association's definition of social phobia (1994) is that it is a marked and persistent fear of one or more social or performance situations – that is, when a person is exposed to either unfamiliar people or possible scrutiny by others. Those with such a phobia fear that they will show anxiety symptoms or act in a way that is humiliating or embarrassing.

Such fears are extremely common, but, because of their very nature (they principally concern being humiliated or embarrassed) they are greatly under-reported, many living with their fears for a lifetime.

The layperson's perception of social phobia as a form of shyness is, in some senses, correct. It is usually, however, much more than simple shyness.

Social phobias usually develop in adolescence, but often only come to the fore when people are required to give talks in public, speak at meetings or be best man at a wedding. The central fears vary considerably. Fears of blushing, sweating or being in any way visibly anxious (such as having a tremor) are very common. In many cases, people use alcohol or drugs to mask their symptoms, which may lead to addictions, with all the serious consequences that follow. People may withdraw from social interaction and become loners, such lifestyles commonly leading to depression.

Many people with agoraphobic fears often also have a marked degree of social phobia and there is considerable overlap between the two conditions. Indeed, social phobias are often accompanied by other mental health problems.

Because people with such phobias tend to avoid social situations, they simply do not get the practice that is required to become socially competent. This lack of practice further inhibits their willingness to enter into interactions with others because of their inability to hold a conversation or perform many of the normal social skills, which compounds the situation. As a result, people with social phobias may appear to have poor social skills because they do not look you in the eye, they stand awkwardly and their facial expression may lack the animation seen in most people. Thus, when it comes to treatment, many social phobics will require some coaching in social skills.

Social phobias respond to the treatment approaches and self-help methods used with simple (specific) phobias. In more severe cases, however, there is a need to treat the accompanying poor self-esteem and low (depressed) mood.

Panic and panic disorder

Being confronted with a phobic object will often lead to panic, but panic attacks may also occur without there being any evidence of phobia. Often, though, panic and phobias are intertwined.

Panic is a very difficult concept to define adequately. One of the problems is that everyone is different and what is experienced as a panic attack by one person may simply be a very high level of anxiety for someone else. Perhaps the best working definition of panic is a condition where, in the mind of the person concerned, the anxiety has become uncontrollable.

The American Psychiatric Association, in its *Diagnostic and Statistical Manual of Mental Disorders* (2000, APA), defined panic as 'a discrete period of intense discomfort in which four or more of the following symptoms developed abruptly and reached a peak within ten minutes'. These symptoms are:

- palpitations, pounding heart or accelerated heart rate
- sweating
- trembling or shaking
- sensations of shortness of breath or smothering

- feelings of choking
- chest pain or discomfort
- nausea or abdominal distress
- feeling dizzy, unsteady, light-headed or faint
- derealization (feelings of unreality) and depersonalization (feelings of being detached from one's self)
- fear of losing control or going crazy
- fear of dying
- numbing or tingling sensations
- chills or hot flushes.

Many people who have panic attacks find that they experience not only 4 of these symptoms but 5, 7 or even all 13 of them! This means that the number of possible combinations of sensations and thoughts that can occur during panic attacks is enormous.

Those who experience panic attacks will know that it is a combination of symptoms such as the above which makes them feel something dreadful is about to happen. The feeling of a loss of control is perhaps the most central preoccupation for most people. Panic attacks can be such a distressing problem that the lives of many become dominated, not by the panic itself but by an anticipation of panic – fear of fear. That fear of fear then begins to form a pattern of preoccupation that may lead people to adapt their lives in a wide variety of ways so as to avoid the attacks occurring.

Some people experience periods when the panics come with some considerable ferocity and then go away for no particular reason. Some of the causes of panic discussed below may give a clue as to why this fluctuating course can occur. During phases when the attacks are common, people very often experience considerable life disruption and if they occur over a long period of time this can have a variety of distressing consequences.

Having panic attacks day in and day out, as is the case for some people, may lead to feelings of dejection and physical exhaustion. Eventually, some may develop depression. Those affected often say that they believe there is no escape from the problem and their lives are not worth living. A significant minority of people with panic disorders may then go on to develop a serious depressive illness that sadly in turn leads to increased susceptibility to panic attacks.

Another possible consequence of long-term panic attacks is for people to develop a reliance on drugs and alcohol. Alcohol seems to provide an instant solution but, if overused, can, of course, lead to serious problems in its own right. A special section of this book is devoted to consideration of the use of alcohol (see Chapter 9). My own research, conducted some years ago, showed that one in five people who have panic attacks and agoraphobia were using alcohol at dangerously high levels. These findings were confirmed by similar studies carried out in the UK and USA.

Spontaneous panic

The psychological and chemical processes that underlie panic attacks are complex. Many people report that they have panic attacks for no apparent reason. Obviously, for some people, there may be a reason for the panic. It may be that a familiar phobia or perhaps something in the environment they were not immediately aware of triggered an attack. It is clear, however, that for some people they just come out of the blue.

Many people who have panic attacks are generally very much more physiologically aroused than the general population and they seem to produce adrenaline more readily than others. Such individuals may be sensitive to other physiological factors, too, that make their arousal system even more vulnerable. For example, being hungry, tired or short of sleep may predispose one to attacks. Some women report that they tend to have panic attacks at certain times in their menstrual cycle and others may be caused by the hormonal changes of the menopause.

Many people report that they are more prone to having apparently spontaneous panic attacks after indulging in alcohol the day before. Likewise, people report that attacks occur in the aftermath of taking illicit drugs, particularly some of the stronger varieties of marijuana (skunk) or ecstasy. It is worth noting that the use of such substances is common and the mental health services see large numbers of people who have panic attacks that are probably largely attributable to drug use.

Agoraphobia with or without panic disorder

The word 'agoraphobia' was originally coined by Carl Westphal, a German neurologist, more than 130 years ago to describe a condition that he had observed in four men. Since then there have been many descriptions of this condition and other names have been attached to it, too.

Agoraphobia is a condition in which anxiety occurs in specific places or situations where people with this condition perceive that escape might be difficult or embarrassing or help might not be readily available. This then leads to them avoiding going out so that they will not have to face the anxiety these places or situations cause, sometimes to such a degree that they become housebound.

Those with agoraphobia have a number of fears, which may include, for example, being away from home, being in a crowd, travelling on public transport, being in a car, standing in a queue, crossing a bridge and so on. Some people only experience panic attacks when confronted with these situations or they anticipate that they will be. Once more a classic pattern of a fear of fear is very common. Others, however, may experience recurrent and unexpected panic attacks that seem to occur spontaneously. For example, sometimes, they may be sitting at home, quietly watching television or undertaking relatively relaxing activities, when the feelings of panic develop, sometimes gradually, sometimes abruptly.

When panic attacks are not linked to a phobic situation and occur at frequent intervals, the condition is sometimes called panic disorder. If the person also suffers agoraphobic fears, then it is sometimes called panic disorder with agoraphobia. To complicate matters further, many people with agoraphobia have fears that are not connected with specific situations, such as public places. Many have health anxieties, so their panic attacks may be triggered by thoughts of illness and death, for example. Often, then, it is possible to trace the source of a panic attack to a specific trigger even when, at first sight, it seems to have occurred for no specific reason. The trigger may be a trivial physical symptom or other bodily sensation or a panic attack may develop after watching a TV film featuring someone with an illness or after reading a newspaper article about someone dying suddenly or contracting a fatal disease.

Agoraphobia usually starts in early adult life with most people saying that it began between the ages of 20 and 30. Sometimes, it starts very suddenly, but it is more usual for the condition to develop in a gradual way, with avoidance behaviour increasing over the course of many years. There is no doubt that agoraphobia can cause wide-ranging restrictions on people's lives and lead to secondary problems, such as poor self-esteem, marital disharmony and depression.

For those with agoraphobia, as for those experiencing panic attacks, often there is a wide range of physical symptoms that they may notice persist, in one shape or form, between panic attacks and exposure to situations away from a secure base. Such symptoms may include palpitations, sweating, a dry mouth, overactivity of the gastrointestinal tract and physically shaking.

Hyperventilation or overbreathing (see Chapter 9) causes additional symptoms, which can be very frightening. These include pins and needles or tingling, yawning, sighing, feeling light-headed and faint, feeling unable to breathe and, in some cases, muscle spasms. These symptoms may lead the person to conclude that he or she is developing a disease such as cancer or multiple sclerosis or is about to collapse and die.

People with agoraphobia may also worry about suddenly losing control, going mad or fainting, running amok, vomiting or becoming incontinent.

Most people know that their fears are irrational. Nevertheless, when the panic attacks come or they are faced with a situation that triggers fear, they are not in control and cannot dispel their fears, so escape from the phobic object or situation seems the only solution.

In addition to specific fears, many agoraphobics would describe themselves as being natural worriers and often anticipating, with anxiety, all kinds of life events. Some people with agoraphobia have other substantial mental health problems, which may include major depressive illnesses, social phobia or OCD.

As many as one in eight of us may have one or two agoraphobic fears. For example, many people avoid travelling on the underground or many other diverse situations because of anxiety. Although, of those referred for treatment, women outnumber men quite substantially, it is known that there are many more men with the problem than the treatment statistics indicate. That is perhaps because, as research shows, men tend to deny or hide their fearfulness much more than women do.

Generalized anxiety states

Most of us know what it feels like to be extremely anxious or apprehensive about an impending family event or a change at work. Generalized anxiety states (sometimes called generalized anxiety disorder or GAD), however, differ from these normal feelings. The term is reserved for those whose excessive anxiety and worry develops to such a degree that it interferes with various aspects of their lives. Such general anxiety commonly accompanies phobias, both simple and complex.

The six central symptoms of generalized anxiety states are:

- restlessness
- being easily fatigued
- difficulty in concentrating or the mind going blank
- irritability
- muscle tension
- sleeplessness.

Generalized anxiety states may cause great impairment of social, occupational and other areas of life. The condition often progresses until people feel downright depressed and dejected.

While some people are, in a sense, born anxious and may have had a lifelong tendency to worry, some generalized anxiety states are triggered by life events. These might be a stressful job, poor relationship or a major life change. Those affected may well have been previously calm and relaxed.

On occasions, people may experience almost continuous, high levels of anxiety. Such a state may not develop into full-blown panic, however. Likewise, although the anxiety may be severe, people often carry on with their normal routine and do not attempt to avoid any specific situations. Anxiety states such as these are known to go through phases and, sometimes, for no apparent reason, periods of relative calm will be experienced.

People with general anxiety often experience great levels of fatigue. As a result, they may be diagnosed as having chronic fatigue syndrome because they feel tired all the time and mention that as being their central complaint. Indeed, it is worth noting that most GPs use the shorthand 'TAT' (for 'tired all the time') to describe this complaint, which is probably one of the commonest symptoms people mention to their GPs. Sadly, many people who are noted as TAT are, in reality, anxious and this is not managed correctly.

Once tests have revealed that nothing abnormal has been detected (NAD in doctors' shorthand), doctors often just shrug their shoulders about what is to be done. Quite often, simple things that you can do are very helpful. Perhaps the most effective is physical exercise, which can now be obtained on prescription from your GP (for more information, see Chapter 9).

Although the treatments described in Part 2 are specifically aimed at the management of phobias and panic, some of the more general advice that I offer regarding exercise, sleep and the use of alcohol may be helpful to those experiencing generalized anxiety states. While there is no magic wand for this or any other anxiety disorder, the recent developments in cognitive therapy and cognitive behaviour therapy (CBT, see Chapter 3) have improved the prospect of great improvements and can make a huge difference to people's lives.

Other related anxiety disorders

There are three conditions in which phobias and phobic behaviour play important parts. These are:

- post-traumatic stress disorder
- obsessive–compulsive disorder
- body dysmorphic disorder.

Post-traumatic stress disorder (PTSD)

Most people think of PTSD as a condition that is related to major disasters, such as the sinking of the Herald of Free Enterprise, the Omagh bombing or the fire at King's Cross station, or else combat situations, such as the wars in Vietnam, Iraq or Afghanistan. In fact, it is very common in the general population, with, it is estimated, up to one in ten of us experiencing some symptoms of PTSD at some time in our lives. For example, nurses, police and fire officers often witness sudden death and various tragic events involving loss of life or mutilation and, as a result, may develop distressing symptoms. Equally it is very common after road traffic accidents and often experienced by victims of violent crime and sexual assaults, too.

The medical definition of post-traumatic stress emphasizes that it has resulted from being exposed to a traumatic event in which the person experienced, witnessed or was confronted with an event or events that involved threatened death, serious injury or a threat to the physical integrity of him- or herself and others. The response usually involves not only a sense of shock and profound fear but also helplessness. The event is remembered in graphic detail, often described as being repeated in slow motion. The definition makes it clear that it occurs not just as a result of being involved directly in or, indeed, suffering a serious injury during, a traumatic event – simply witnessing one or thinking that you are about to be killed or seriously injured can be sufficient to cause the problem.

PTSD comprises a range of symptoms. Very often people experience recurrent and intrusive recollections of the event, often in dreams but sometimes in the form of visual flashbacks that occur while they are awake. Any confrontation with things that remind them of the original event – for example, driving close to the site of an accident – may cause considerable distress, which, in turn, leads to avoidance. They may experience a numbing of their general responses and show a markedly diminished interest in their usual activities. People with this disorder very often complain of feeling detached or estranged from others and may see no future for themselves. Other symptoms include sleep disturbance, irritability or anger and finding it hard to concentrate. At the same time, they may become constantly aware of any possible danger in their environment.

The commonest symptom of PTSD is anxiety that is all-pervasive, coupled with avoidance of many varied situations. As is the case with most phobias, the anxiety and avoidance grow, very often leading to greater depression. It is therefore very important that the phobic elements of PTSD are treated (see the Useful contacts section (p. 106) for some sources of help). I would also suggest reading Dr Claudia Herbert's excellent book (see the References section on p. 109) and visiting NICE's website (at: <www.nice.org.uk/guidance/CG26>) to read through its guidelines for a comprehensive account of what treatment is advised.

Obsessive–compulsive disorder (OCD)

OCD is mentioned here because it is one of the anxiety states that often leads to attacks of panic and avoidance behaviour.

OCD can take many forms but essentially consists of either intrusive, repetitive and distressing thoughts or compulsions, such as washing hands frequently or checking or repeating an activity. More often than not, people with OCD experience both of these phenomena and some of the commonest obsessions are linked to a fear of dirt or germs or of simply doing things 'wrong' or imperfectly. A dirt and germs phobia can lead to people repeatedly washing their hands, sometimes taking hours to ensure that their hands are perfectly clean. They are, however, never happy with the end result and the interminable vicious circle commences again.

Sometimes people are afraid of losing control, which is often linked to obsessional and intrusive thoughts regarding the consequences of that happening. As a result, even the kindest, gentlest person may begin to worry about a loss of control that may lead to him or her committing a violent act or else a deeply religious person may fear shouting out a blasphemy or obscenity in church. Needless to say, such fears are groundless and these things never happen, but the people concerned are often completely overwhelmed by their anxieties and depression is very common in the severest cases.

OCD is a common condition, affecting about 3 to 4 per cent of the population, and many people with phobias and panic disorder are also affected by OCD.

On a more optimistic note, the cognitive behavioural treatments developed for OCD over the last 20 years have brought real hope for those affected and treatment approaches are being developed all the time. This condition can be helped by both professional and self-help methods and some of the treatment principles described in Chapter 3 can be applied to OCD with a good chance of success.

Body dysmorphic disorder (BDD)

Body dysmorphic disorder is a relatively new term. It was coined by the American Psychiatric Association in 1994 to describe people who have a preoccupation with an imagined defect in their appearance. It is also applied when people have an actual slight physical anomaly and become disproportionately preoccupied with it.

One difficulty with carrying out research in this area is that people with this condition are very reluctant to come forward for interview and those who do often have great trouble providing comprehensive information about their difficulties, usually because of a great sense of embarrassment. There is universal acceptance, however, that this condition results in very significant social and psychological handicaps.

BDD usually starts in adolescence and the studies that have been carried out have all found that people with this condition have difficulty in forming and maintaining social relationships. The condition is often associated with social phobia and more general obsessional thinking. We also know from research that up to a quarter of people with BDD have attempted suicide. Many try to change their perceived body imperfection by having plastic surgery or camouflage it with make-up. Generally, however, these do not help and, in fact, often make the problem worse.

Over the years I have seen dozens of people with this condition. One of the striking features is that, although they may often come across as shy or very shy, they are, like most anxious people, otherwise very normal. Many hold down responsible jobs but, at the same time, often suffer enormous handicaps because of their avoidance of social situations and the psychological distress they experience.

BDD has been studied by NICE, resulting in it issuing guidance (available online at: <www.nice.org.uk/guidance/CG31>). The guidance recommends psychological treatments (CBT) and medication – high dose selective serotonin reuptake inhibitors (SSRIs), such as fluoxetine (in the form of Prozac, for example), are the commonest drugs used. While the results of such treatments are encouraging, in my experience many people are resistant to being treated and very few report a complete, or near complete, recovery. A good treatment outcome for BDD therefore usually means that the distress and handicap caused by the condition is reduced by about 70 per cent. Thus, for most people, it is a lifelong condition. I came across a lady in her late seventies whose condition – although it has slightly improved over the decades – still causes a considerable degree of psychological distress and social handicap.

Children's fears and phobias

The first point to be made is that children have many more fears and phobias than adults and often, when they are afraid, their emotions are intensely felt. Nevertheless, their fears and phobias can also come and go quickly and for no apparent reason.

One of the most important pieces of advice I give to parents is to practice 'watchful waiting'. When parents become aware that their child has a particular problem, the first response is sometimes to seek help and treatment. In many cases, this is unnecessary as the fears and phobias will often decline over time. It is, however, worth mentioning that the watchful waiting advice should be accompanied by a sensible approach to gradually increasing exposure of the child to the source of the fear or phobia. This is achieved by helping the child face whatever it is in graduated doses of difficulty, with an important emphasis on him or her seeing someone else confront the same object or situation. Thus, for example, if a child had a fear of dogs (which is very common), it would be worthwhile seeking out places where he or she might see dogs being taken for a walk in a family setting so that the child could watch others happily playing with their family pets. It is usually very unhelpful to protect children from their phobic objects or situations as this may well make the problem much worse.

It is quite normal for preschool children to have a fear of animals, sleeping alone, loud noises and so on. Around the time children start school, they develop a more acute imagination and at this point they may come to fear ghosts and monsters. Most parents will, however, be familiar with children who love to be scared and will often make the request, 'Please read me that scary story.'

Most children go through periods of greater attachment to one or other of their parents or may take an irrational dislike to even close relatives and friends. Once more, an approach based on not reinforcing the behaviour is wise and the feared person should simply carry on as usual until the fear goes away.

In their early school years, children become more able to think in the abstract and about the future. Thus, they gradually become more aware of death, disaster and war. The age that preoccupations with these subjects begins varies considerably from child to child, but with the enormously expanded access to all kinds of the media, it may be that such fears become apparent at an earlier age than used to be the case. The difficulty here is that, for very young children who are only just beginning to develop the ability to think and reason in an abstract way, it can be difficult to explain what may happen in the future.

Different fears and phobias can start at different ages. Fears relating to animals generally start in young children and, although many of these phobias will simply disappear, some will persist into adult life. Social phobias – fears of other people or social situations – tend to start in the period just before puberty. Fears of enclosed spaces, agoraphobia and the like usually begin in the late teenage years.

The ways in which fear manifests in children is different from the process in adults. Children experience fear differently in terms of its intensity and the sensation of it, in both physical and mental aspects. Some children may express their anxiety outwardly by complaining of a tummy ache or a headache, while others will simply become very withdrawn and uncommunicative.

Professionals who treat children generally have a greater understanding of child development than most health professionals who usually treat adults – therapists tend to treat either adults or children, but not both. There are occasions when, because of a shortage of resources, therapists who treat adults will see children. Whatever the case, therapists should have some specific experience and training so that they can put the child's fears into the correct developmental context for him or her.

Perhaps the most commonly described fear in children is school phobia – sometimes called school refusal. This topic has become the source of great controversy because there is often an inability to distinguish between different forms of the behaviour associated with it. Sometimes children fear school because they are anxious about being separated from their parents and may become worried that they will never see their mother or father or siblings again. Other children can be afraid of the school situation itself and fear the teacher or other children.

School refusal commonly occurs after being away from school for a period of time, perhaps after an illness, but often after the long summer holiday. Sometimes school phobias develop when a child changes school.

Refusing to go to school may be a problem that is made worse by parental attention and, while no one wishes to see a child upset or distressed, making a great fuss of him or her because he or she feels anxious at school and, in a sense, rewarding this behaviour with additional attention, gifts and so on, may simply reinforce it. For the parent involved in this situation, how to handle it is a real conundrum.

Tragically, some children may not go to school because of anxiety on the part of their parents. In my career I have seen mothers and one or two fathers who have a fear of being on their own and so have kept their children at home for company. Such situations are very difficult to resolve and will often require psychiatric input for the parent involved as well as help for the child.

Sometimes, children develop fears that they find very difficult to disclose to anyone. Examples of such fears include concerns about undressing in front of other children before swimming or games lessons, being bullied by others or, more commonly than one would think, of fainting, vomiting and incontinence. Sometimes children are unable to put their fear into words, simply saying, 'I feel afraid' or that they don't feel safe at school.

I have here provided only a brief outline of the nature of children's fears and phobias. This is a complex subject, about which health professionals and teachers often disagree, so it is easy to see why sometimes it is difficult to distinguish between a real fear or phobia and simply not wanting to go to school. Truanting behaviour is, of course, another subject and may have its own psychological and emotional roots, not necessarily connected with fears or phobias.

Unfortunately, we seem, overall, to know less about children's fears and phobias than adults' and child and adolescent mental health services are under such enormous pressure that help is not readily available, in the public, NHS or independent sectors.

Conclusion

This chapter has described a wide variety of anxiety states and phobias as well as highlighting the kinds of physical symptoms that they may cause. It has shown us that phobias and avoidance behaviours are very common and can cause considerable disruption to people's lives, undoubtedly affecting their general well-being and quality of life. No one is immune so it is possible for anybody to be affected by one or other of these disorders at some time. For some of us it will be a passing phase; for others it may be a continuing distressing and disabling condition.

The next chapter describes how these conditions arise and explores the possible causes, before I move on, in the rest of the book, to consider how they can be managed by either professional or self-help means.

2

Causes of anxiety and phobias

Before considering the issue of causation, we need first to talk about adrenaline – the hormone of the fight or flight response.

Adrenaline

Adrenaline, also called epinephrine, is a hormone produced by the adrenal glands. There are two of these glands, one sitting on top of each kidney.

The function of adrenaline is to prepare the body for action and activity in response to dangerous situations and so on. The hormone does this by increasing the supply of oxygen and glucose to the brain and muscles and, at the same time, suppresses other non-essential bodily processes. Thus, adrenaline increases respiration, heart rate and blood pressure and also dilates the pupils. The pupils dilate so that we can see as much as possible of the environment. The heart rate may double and blood pressure may rise to very high levels. Adrenaline produces a number of other changes in the body, including the primitive response of causing the muscles at the base of our hairs to contract, leading to that 'hair standing up on the back of your neck' feeling we associate with being scared or danger. In animals this response to danger makes the animal look fiercer so can help them to scare off predators.

All these physical processes that result from the release of adrenaline enable the body to function in an optimum state. While many people worry about the various physical changes that follow a release of adrenaline, the body – even in people with serious illnesses – can withstand the effects, no problem. Indeed, adrenaline is injected in emergencies when someone needs to be resuscitated. When the body is under the influence of high levels of adrenaline, the heart muscle is probably working at its optimum efficiency.

People are concerned about the long-term effects of the fight or flight response, also called the stress reaction, but the evidence for anxiety in itself shortening life or causing various illnesses is quite limited. There is even some evidence that anxious people live longer than their relaxed fellows.

While it is quite true that prolonged exposure to stress may adversely affect blood pressure and the immune system, there is no clear evidence that even those who live with extreme levels of panic have a shorter lifespan. In studies that link stress and anxiety with heart attacks and reduced life expectancy, one needs to take into account that such individuals may also engage in unhealthy behaviours, such as drinking too much alcohol or smoking. They may also not engage in healthy behaviours, such as taking regular aerobic exercise or eating a healthy diet. When these factors are taken into consideration, the evidence for panic attacks and high levels of anxiety causing major health problems diminishes.

What causes anxiety and phobias?

The simple answer is this: nobody can really provide a definitive account of how anxiety and phobias arise.

There is a great deal of research that helps us to see how some factors may be implicated in the causation of these conditions, but the truth is that there is no single all-embracing theory. Some psychologists and physiologists say that they have the answer – in my career I have heard such proclamations many times. In the course of time an answer may come, but I think that the only certainty is there will never be a single comprehensive theory that covers everyone and their particular condition.

Various new technologies have provided major advances in many areas. For example, we can now see the brain much more clearly than previously when we only had conventional X-rays. Magnetic resonance imaging (MRI) scans can provide images of the working brain. We also have radioactive isotopes that can be used to detect the chemical changes occurring during panic attacks and genetic technologies that promise a great deal.

Brain imaging using MRI scans have allowed researchers to examine the brains of people while they perform various tasks or are exposed to some anxiety-provoking situations. Such research has shown clearly that certain areas of the brain are implicated in anxiety and seems to suggest that the brains of those who experience states of anxiety may differ in subtle ways from those of people without anxiety states. There is now a strong probability that a great deal of anxiety may be genetically determined (for example, scientists are fairly certain that there is a substantial genetic component to panic disorder, agoraphobia and obsessive–compulsive disorder) and, in the decades to come, treatments based on DNA technology may be developed. It is impossible to predict, however, how much the children of people with these disorders are at risk of developing these conditions.

Research also seems to confirm the long-held view that most people with anxiety are, in some way, biologically predisposed to reacting in a more marked way physiologically than other people, simply pumping out more adrenaline. This predisposition may combine with other psychological and social factors occurring during childhood and, later in life, a fear or a phobia may develop.

Sometimes, however, when I listen to the history of someone with an anxiety disorder, it becomes clear that it started after a specific trauma. For example, the person may have been involved in an accident or trapped in a lift or else it may have developed as a response to a sudden bereavement or a separation. In such cases, the person may or may not have previously had a predisposition to anxiety.

What is interesting is that people who suffer similar traumas often react in very different ways, some developing problems that may persist in the long term while others endure their experiences with no particular difficulty. A partial explanation of this comes from cognitive psychologists, who have shown that learning to react in an anxious way is, for some people, the most important factor in the way their anxiety develops. This does not apply in every case, which highlights once more the tremendous variation that exists in the causation of these conditions.

Finally, social factors are of great importance in the way that anxiety states evolve. Some years ago I conducted some research on sex roles and agoraphobia. Not surprisingly, this work confirmed the long-held view that women are more predisposed to developing conditions such as agoraphobia than men because of their general social roles, dependence on others perhaps being more acceptable in women than men. Furthermore, some male spouses may actually encourage their partners to increase their dependency on them. My research also showed, however, that many more women than men attend for treatment, but there are many men who will not admit to their fearfulness. While these men do not come for treatment, they often seek a solution to their problem by turning to alcohol.

Other social factors that cause an increased vulnerability to anxiety are, understandably, poverty, social isolation and unemployment. Yet another social dimension that has been extensively explored in relation to depression is the role of social support. George Brown and Tirrill Harris (1978), two researchers at the Institute of Psychiatry and Bedford College in London, investigated this and found that those women who had close confiding relationships were much less vulnerable than those without such support structures. Research into anxiety disorders indicates that the same is true for these conditions as for depression. The acknowledged very positive effects of social support are an excellent reason for encouraging people to get in touch with self-help organizations, which may be able to offer such support.

Conclusion

We have seen how anxiety, panic and phobias develop in different ways in different people. There is clear evidence that biological, psychological and social factors are all important in their causation. The precise contributions each of these factors make, however, is still far from clear. It may be that, in conditions such as panic disorder, in one person it is primarily caused by biological factors (such as an excessive production of adrenaline), while in another, even though they both experience the same symptoms, it is a childhood trauma. Often, though, we will never know the precise causes.

3

Treatments

There has been a very welcome move to recognize that the treatments offered to people with anxiety disorders and who have panic attacks should be based on sound evidence from research and delivered by trained practitioners. In turn, as mentioned above, NICE regularly issues guidance on the best treatments for various problems, both physical and mental.

Despite such a climate, it is clear that many, if not most, members of the general public are still unaware of which treatments are best and are forever being confused by misleading reports in the media telling of the next wonder treatment or distressed by scare stories that panic attacks lead to heart attacks.

One of the other issues to address is the point of view held by a sizeable proportion of the population, and indeed some of the professional community, that treatments with a strong evidence base are not the only effective interventions for panic and phobias. While in this book I recognize that more general approaches, such as relaxation and breathing exercises, a good diet and aerobic exercise, are all of considerable importance, I have concentrated my attention on treatments with a strong evidence base. I appreciate that there is an array of alternative treatments available and, although space does not allow an exploration of alternative treatments here, I recognize that some people who undergo alternative treatments do seem to benefit from them.

I shall now discuss the two central approaches to treating phobias and panic, the effectiveness of which is supported by an enormous amount of research evidence. These are:

- cognitive behaviour therapy
- medication.

I will also discuss some other treatment approaches.

Cognitive behaviour therapy (CBT)

CBT did not exist when I started my professional career some 40 years ago. What did exist at that time was behaviour therapy. Cognitive behaviour therapy, now familiar to millions, grew out of behaviour therapy and has developed into perhaps the most important and certainly the best-researched form of psychological therapy in modern times.

How CBT developed

Behaviour therapy developed as a result of the work of experimental psychologists who studied human behaviour and came to understand that many fears can be seen as learned responses.

In the field of anxiety disorders, behaviour therapy was developed in the 1950s by a number of individuals, but one man – Dr Joseph Wolpe – stands out as a luminary. Joe Wolpe developed a technique called 'systematic desensitization' to deal with phobias.

Systematic desensitization involves the person with a fear imagining the phobic object, such as spiders, and learning a response that is incompatible with anxiety about it. Thus, Wolpe taught people to think about their phobic object, but at the same time engage in deep, physical relaxation.

The original form of systematic desensitization was a very prolonged therapy based on the idea of a hierarchy – that is, a long list of images connected with the feared object, but arranged in graduated levels of difficulty. Thus, in the case of a fear of spiders, at the bottom of the hierarchy might be having a little money spider in a sealed glass jar some 30 metres away from you and the top might be having a tarantula placed on the palm of your hand. In between there might be 100 steps.

Wolpe's technique of systematic desensitization involved dealing with each step in the hierarchy by teaching the phobic person to relax and, only when he or she could fully relax with that particular step did he move on to the next step. The technique was, therefore, very time-consuming and took many months, but proved very effective.

Before systematic desensitization, the only treatment available for phobias was medication, which often had dreadful side effects, or years of psychoanalysis. In those days (the 1950s), psychoanalysis was a very scarce commodity and, used in its traditional form, involved three sessions a week for three to five years. The therapy sessions explored a person's childhood and the deep 'unconsciousness'.

When systematic desensitization was first introduced, the psychoanalysts of the time protested and said that phobias were caused by deep unconscious conflicts (often of a sexual nature). The analysts warned that when phobias were cured by systematic desensitization, another phobia would arise – so-called symptom substitution. Over the past 50 years or thereabouts, research has proved the psychoanalysts to be mostly incorrect.

Systematic desensitization using the imagination developed over time into the therapy of graduated exposure in real life and modern-day behaviour therapy came of age about 35 years ago. When I began my training in the use of behaviour therapy, it was used for, perhaps, 10 per cent of people who came to psychiatric outpatient clinics. Most of my work at that time was targeted at fears, phobias, obsessions and compulsions. Behaviour therapy for these conditions entailed a process of exposure in graduated levels of difficulty, with the emphasis being on helping people to stay in the phobic situation and teaching them that prolonged exposure would lead to the anxiety eventually abating and nothing dreadful happening.

Although there were many successes with this approach, many clinicians began to realize that dramatic changes in behaviour had very positive effects on thinking, but an anxious mindset often prevented recovery. Thus, approximately 25 years ago, cognitive therapy for fears and phobias, obsessions and compulsions began to be developed in earnest.

We began to understand that, while graduated exposure is a very powerful form of treatment, it is important to try and help people change how they think about their phobias and anxieties – they need to work on all their mental processes, including thoughts, images and memories. Thus, over time, CBT developed into the very broad treatment approach that is used today for a very wide range of mental health problems.

My friends and colleagues Rob Willson and Rhena Branch, in their excellent book, *Cognitive Behavioural Therapy for Dummies*, have very helpfully defined CBT as an approach that is a combination of the scientific, philosophical and behavioural. All of these elements together form a comprehensive approach to understanding and overcoming common psychological problems.

Rhena and Rob define the scientific part of CBT in two ways. First, they state that the therapy has been tested in scientific studies, using the same randomized controlled trials format that is used to test the effects of drugs and surgical treatment. Second, they explain that CBT also uses a scientific approach in terms of the way in which the therapist and client work together as the thoughts that the person has in connection with his or her fears and phobias are treated as theories and hunches that need to be tested. Thus, for example, if you believe that you will collapse and die if you go into a supermarket and you are overcome by anxiety about that, it is a thought (belief) that needs to be put to the test. This can be done by a process of discussion, but then, most importantly, by actually entering the feared situation and testing out the theory for yourself.

CBT also recognizes that people have a very wide range of values and beliefs about themselves, the world, other people and the future. In this, CBT is certainly person-centred. Therapists set out to help people achieve their own treatment goals, not those of the therapist or others.

CBT is a process that emphasizes behaviour. Therefore, in over-coming phobias, people change their behaviour by gradually facing something that has previously been avoided. More recently, in the treatment of depression, the emphasis of CBT has been on the 'activa-tion' of the individual, recognizing that one of the central features of depression is inactivity and withdrawal from the world. This is because it is known that such withdrawal leads to further problems, with depression and so on, so activity is an essential target of a treatment programme.

The central treatment technique in CBT for phobias and panic is exposure therapy. This therapy is based on principles that have been around for literally thousands of years and, as Isaac Marks has pointed out on a number of occasions, philosophers such as Joseph Locke (in his *An Essay Concerning Human Understanding* in 1690) advocated exposure as the central method for overcoming a phobia. Indeed, even Sigmund Freud, the archetypal advocate of psychoanalytic treat-ments, said in several of his works that, once the analysis has worked, the person needs to face the fear! (This is a liberal paraphrasing of his advice.)

Twenty years ago, exposure treatments were usually administered by a therapist who helped people to face their fears. Indeed, I can remember spending 20 or 30 hours with people with agoraphobia on the London underground, staying with them until their anxiety reduced or spending many hours in shopping centres helping people to be able to face crowds and queues. It has been shown over the years, however, that, as long as people are helped to make the initial entry into the phobic situation, such intensive therapeutic assistance is unnecessary. Although it is important to explain the exposure principle (that anxiety reduces if you stay in the phobic situation and gradually diminishes with repeated exposures), people may ask a family member or friend to help them keep to their exposure routine consistently over a longer period of time. For more details as to how to conduct exposure therapy, see Chapter 7.

In CBT, it is essential that therapists and clients work together as a team. CBT is a therapy that is collaborative and inclusive. In order to be collaborative, therapists often need to educate their clients. Such education may, for example, include explanations of the nature of anxiety, how adrenaline affects the body, whether or not anxiety is harmful to health, whether or not panic attacks will inevitably lead to a heart attack and so on. Education also includes helping people to understand that avoiding situations giving rise to fear will only strengthen the fear itself.

Where possible, therapists should set out to help clients understand their condition, as much as they can. They should also provide information about which websites to visit and so on. Therapists must be honest about the effectiveness of treatment. To this end, it is helpful that we now have the NICE guidance on the effectiveness of various treatment approaches that may be passed on to the people we treat. Although the guidance available on various topics includes versions written in non-technical language, the NICE website also gives references for published papers and so on for anyone who wishes to explore one or more of them in greater detail.

The availability of huge amounts of information has caused many, including doctors and therapists, a great deal of anxiety because clients can sometimes know as much, if not more, than they do! Indeed, it is certainly not unknown for people who have conducted their own research on the Internet to ask me questions, such as, 'If 70 per cent of people respond to CBT for my problem, what about the other 30 per cent? Is it more or less likely that I will be in this 30 per cent rather than the 70 per cent?' Alternatively, 'Of the 70 per cent who get better, how many are totally cured?' All these questions, of course, mean that therapists need to provide honest answers. Sometimes, that means simply saying, 'I don't know'. Then, of course, the therapist has to go away and find out. Sometimes, though, there is no answer. Whatever the situation, if therapists are to work in a truly collaborative way with people in their treatment, they cannot simply tell people what to do.

Access to CBT

While it is true that there are now, literally, thousands of research papers that tell professionals about the effectiveness of CBT for fears and phobias and, in the UK, the NHS proudly proclaims through NICE that such treatment is recommended, the common experience of most people is that they have enormous difficulty accessing professional help. In this section, however, I will attempt to explain what professional help may be available and what you need to look for in a therapist.

The first port of call for anyone with a health problem should be his or her GP. It is pleasing to know that GPs are increasingly becoming familiar with the nature of fears and phobias and there are effective treatments available that do not involve swallowing pills. So, if you need help, it is worth discussing your problem with your GP. I would, however, suggest that you first try a self-help programme, such as that outlined in Part 2. By this, I mean that you should attempt to stick to a programme and carry it out in a systematic manner for at least three weeks and possibly up to three months.

Initially, your GP may refer you to a psychiatrist. If so, it does not mean that the GP simply thinks you are mad or require admission to hospital. Sometimes, GPs prefer to do this, particularly if the psychiatrist in question has an interest in fears and phobias. The psychiatrist may then make a referral to a suitable therapist. Therapists come from a range of backgrounds and, in the UK, there is a small number of psychiatrists who have received additional training in CBT and carry out a limited number of treatments themselves. That said, extensive training in CBT is not common among psychiatrists and even those who have had such training may not be able to see very many people because of other demands on their time.

Establishing that your therapist has reasonable training in CBT is often a daunting task, but there are some simple things you can do that will greatly improve your chances of finding out.

Anyone offering CBT whose work is of a reasonable standard will be registered with either the British Psychological Society (<www.bps.org.uk>) or the British Association for Behavioural and Cognitive Psychotherapies (<www.babcp.com>). Both these organizations have online search facilities and you can simply look up a therapist's name. In addition, it is worth noting that the Health Professions Council (<www.hpc-uk.org>) is the third government regulatory body besides the General Medical Council (which regulates doctors) and the Nursing and Midwifery Council (which regulates nurses and midwives). The Health Professions Council registers over 200,000 professionals from 14 professions. In August 2009, it took over regulatory responsibility for the British Psychological Society, so you can find practising psychologists on the registers at both websites.

To complicate matters somewhat, although many CBT therapists come from one of the health professions, some do not, but may have a degree in psychology (not clinical psychology) and have taken additional courses to qualify as a cognitive behaviour therapist. At the time of writing, the Health Professions Council is attempting to develop a regulatory framework for psychotherapists and counsellors (who both offer a range of psychological treatments), but I am sure that this will be an uphill task. For some 30 years there have been attempts to regulate the work of psychotherapists and counsellors, but various problems have emerged that have prevented them from coming about. As a note of caution, literally anyone can put up a brass plate on the front of an impressive-looking office and practise as a therapist or counsellor, charging whatever he or she wants. Indeed, many thousands of people across the UK are receiving therapy from people who lack any credible qualifications.

The major problem at present is that the number of therapists available to deliver CBT in the UK is still woefully small. It is unfortunately not uncommon to see people who have been referred for NHS treatment for their phobia having to wait many months just for an assessment. In some cases, to compound the problem, following that assessment they may then be placed on a waiting list for treatment, which, again, means that it is several months before they receive it. When treatment is offered, it is sometimes limited to six to eight sessions. That may suffice for some problems, but is grossly insufficient for the treatment of some complex fears and phobias.

In 2006, the UK government began to improve access to and increase the quantity of psychological therapies for adults of working age, announcing that many millions would be made available to fund the programme Improving Access to Psychological Therapies (IAPT). The current aim is to have more than 3600 newly trained therapists by 2010/2011. The government argues that this will allow literally hundreds of thousands more people to have access to treatment than in the past.

Therapists trained under the programme fall into two categories. First, there are the so-called low-intensity therapists. These therapists have received some training, but much less than a fully accredited CBT therapist. Low-intensity therapists might be able to help with simple anxiety states, phobias and depression.

The second category is high-intensity therapists, who generally have considerable experience and training in providing psychological therapies. Such therapists will generally be clinical psychologists, counselling psychologists, nurse therapists, primary care counsellors and other qualified mental health professionals.

Although everyone would agree that there is a need to train more therapists and for effective psychological treatments to be more readily available, the IAPT programme appears to have a number of problems in terms of its implementation. Understandably within an organization as large as the NHS, practical and bureaucratic problems have prevented it from being implemented effectively and there is still some controversy among mental health professionals about the type, quantity and level of training required.

As in all matters concerning public services, cost is a central issue. Given the current economic downturn, it is difficult to see how the original optimism about this programme will be borne out in reality. Nevertheless, it is encouraging that real money appears to have gone into the training of an essential workforce. Self-help is, however, still required and it also needs to be said that the IAPT programme has, from the very beginning, emphasized that, if it is to succeed, it is necessary to continue with efforts to deliver self-help programmes to those who need them.

Those with fears and phobias should always be aware that they have a right to be treated by a properly qualified therapist within the NHS. My advice to those in need is this: you have to continually emphasize your right to treatment and quote the NICE guidelines that recommend treatment as often as possible.

With regard to the main self-help organizations in the UK, note that the more widely used ones all have networks of highly trained health professionals with specialist backgrounds in treating fears and phobias at their disposal. For example, at No Panic, all of the sources and interventions provided are subject to scrutiny by a very wide range of professional advisers and, wherever possible, interventions are chosen based on the best evidence for their effectiveness.

Computerized cognitive behaviour therapy (CCBT)

CCBT is now a treatment approved by NICE and has been demonstrated to benefit people who have various fears, phobias and obsessive–compulsive disorder.

Two decades ago, Professor Isaac Marks began to develop a computerized form of his self-help book *Living with Fear*. He was able to see, as early as the 1970s, that, in the future, the shortage of CBT therapists would become an increasing problem for the NHS. Because of his research, Professor Marks had at that time become convinced that self-help was an effective method for treating fears and phobias and so began to develop a computerized version of his book. He also foresaw that people would require some professional input and need education in not only how to use the computer programs (bearing in mind that 20 years ago most people did not have access to a computer) but also in the form of support and encouragement to pursue the self-help programme.

Marks, although at the forefront of the movement to computerize CBT, was not alone. Many others in the UK and across the world identified that computers could be an effective means for treating literally millions of people. The story of how CCBT has developed is fascinating and has been the subject of many research articles, chapters and books.

Today, CCBT is available on the NHS and NICE recommends Fearfighter as the preferred package. Local health trusts purchase a licence to use Fearfighter and make it available in GPs' surgeries and other convenient locations. Normally, a health professional introduces you to the package and then you systematically work through – over a period of 6 to 12 weeks – a step-by-step self-help programme. It is, in many ways, similar to the steps set out in the self-help programme in Part 2, but, in addition to the computer package you would have some access to professional help.

There are now several other computer programs to buy as packages or via the Internet to load on to your PC that are similar to Fearfighter. The quality of these programs does vary somewhat, however, and only Fearfighter has been approved by the NHS for use with phobias.

Some other programs have also been developed for people who have depression that are available on the Internet and several are free. One such program, from Australia (<www.moodgym.anu.edu.au>), has been shown in a number of research studies to be very helpful for people with mild to moderate depression and may be of some assistance to people with fears and phobias who are also depressed. The research evidence emphasizes that MoodGYM is effective on its own but, for maximum effect, probably needs the person to have some contact with a mental health professional. Three years ago I reviewed this program and others on behalf of the NHS and have used it in my own clinical work. There are some drawbacks but, overall, for anyone with some measure of depression it is well worth a try.

The NHS, via NICE, also recommends another package for the treatment of depression, Beating the Blues (<www.beatingtheblues.co.uk>). Like Fearfighter, it is available in GPs' surgeries and other convenient locations.

There have been several other developments using computer technology. For example, in the US and the UK computer-generated virtual reality has been used for the treatment of phobias. This involves you wearing a head-mounted display unit and then being presented with a computer-generated 'world' that changes naturally as you move your head and/or body. Some such units also include gloves to allow additional contact with the virtual world. In this way, interaction with a virtual environment becomes possible.

There is plentiful evidence that such treatments are effective in enabling people to overcome phobias. This is obviously a very good way of graduating exposure to the phobic object or situation and can help to prepare people so that they can then face the real phobic object with much less difficulty.

This technology is probably most beneficial for situations that are not readily accessible or occur in a random way. For example, people with thunder and lightning phobias could be exposed to virtual thunder storms, those with a fear of flying could be prepared before embarking on a trip in a real plane and people who dislike enclosed spaces or crowds could travel on a virtual underground train or visit a busy virtual shopping centre.

The major drawbacks to this treatment are the high initial cost of the equipment and therapists would need to be trained to be able to use it.

There are now a number of other developments that may assist people with anxiety and I am sure more will follow. The introduction of palm-top programs, stressbusters via your TV remote, a range of fitness programmes and the like are to be welcomed. The benefits are that they can be a source of highly accessible and effective interventions, but, perhaps more importantly, they serve to show people that at some time anxiety will rear its head in the vast majority of the population.

Medication

It is true to say that drug treatments for panic and phobias are as old as history. Indeed, the commonest remedy for all forms of anxiety has been the drug alcohol. It is still is very frequently used by those with phobias and panic and can, of course, lead to very serious problems.

Tranquillizers

The twentieth century saw an evolution in the treatment of various anxiety states with drugs, moving from opiates (morphine-like drugs) in the early part of the century to bromides and barbiturates. Some of these drugs were effective, at least in the short term, in reducing anxiety but, to say the least, they were toxic and their use accounted for huge levels of addiction and many deaths.

The 1960s saw the widespread introduction of benzodiazepines (drugs such as Valium and Ativan) and, by the 1980s, some 27 million prescriptions for tranquillizers were issued each year in the UK. Their use was so common that it was estimated 1 woman in 3 over 40 had a regular prescription for a Valium-type drug in any single year.

The most commonly prescribed drug then and now is diazepam (the tradename of which is Valium), although several other varieties of benzodiazepines (such as Ativan and Xanax) have also been prescribed in large quantities. Benzodiazepines have also been used as sleeping tablets.

Essentially these drugs all work in the same way, although some are more sleep-inducing than others. The marketing for them was accompanied by many reports of their effectiveness and, indeed, as short-term medications, they certainly calm the nerves. Similarly, the benzodiazepine group of drugs are generally very safe and excellent when used to help people cope with dentistry and minor surgical procedures.

The great difficulty with these drugs, however, is that they quickly lead to addiction and their beneficial effect on anxiety wears off after a few dozen doses. Thus, the current treatment guidelines suggest that, if these drugs are to be prescribed, they are only to be used for a very short period (no more than 28 days) and in as low a dose as possible. It is therefore reasonable for someone to be prescribed a very short course of medication to deal with very distressing life events. Drugs such as diazepam are also used quite effectively for certain medical complaints. For example, diazepam – which is probably effective in treating anxiety because it relaxes the muscles – is often used as a short-term measure for dealing with back pain and spasms and may be used to relax those who have high blood pressure.

In terms of treating panic and phobias, these drugs are not to be recommended. I do believe, however, that for some people with very specific fears, such as flying, who do not need to face their phobic situation very often and for whom psychological treatment might be impractical, the use of small amounts of drugs like diazepam to, in this case, get you off the ground is not altogether a bad thing. Although some of my colleagues may raise their eyebrows at such a recommendation, I perhaps need to remind them that they might generally recommend that some of the 40 per cent of people who become anxious when taking a trip on an aeroplane have a gin and tonic at the airport! It seems to me that one or two doses of diazepam, taken once a year, may be less harmful than the proverbial Dutch courage, even if it is condoned by society at large.

One of the great problems now is that there are still many people who were prescribed benzodiazepine tranquillizers before we knew what we know now, have been taking them for many years and are clearly addicted. These unfortunate individuals are in the position of taking drugs that provide no real benefit in terms of their condition, yet may cause side effects such as drowsiness, a deadening of feelings and emotions, weight gain and memory problems. If they were to stop taking these medications abruptly, however, they would suffer terrible withdrawal symptoms and, in extreme circumstances, major health problems such as seizures. To withdraw from these drugs safely often takes months, if not years. A simple rule of thumb is that it takes at least one month of withdrawal for every year that the person has been on the drug. Thus, it is still not uncommon for me to be monitoring people who were first prescribed these medications in the 1960s.

Over the years, a number of self-help groups have grown up for people addicted to tranquillizers and the work they do is invaluable. If you have a tranquillizer problem, see if there is a group in your area listed on the Internet. One of the very active groups in the UK, located in Lancashire, is Beat the Benzos (see the Useful contacts section (p. 106) for details).

Antidepressants

If you look at treatment guidelines for panic and phobia, you will see that the use of antidepressant medications is recommended.

There are various antidepressants that are marketed for the treatment of anxiety. The main group of drugs used now is the selective serotonin reuptake inhibitors (SSRIs). These have a variety of names, such as Prozac (fluoxetine), Seroxat (paroxetine), Cipramil (citalopram), Cipralex (escitalopram). There are also drugs related to SSRIs that are prescribed, such as Cymbalta (duloxetine) and Efexor (venlafaxine).

It is interesting to note that our reliance on medication as a first-line treatment for anxiety states is increasing over the years. There is plentiful evidence that, while prescriptions of the Valium family of drugs (the benzodiazepines – see p. 55) have greatly reduced from the 27 million per year in the UK in 1987, at the same time there has been a great increase in the number of prescriptions of SSRIs for anxiety states. At the present time, more than 30 million prescriptions for SSRIs are issued in the UK each year and 170 million in the USA, at a cost in the UK of approximately £3 billion. While the majority of these are prescribed for depression, a very significant proportion of them go to people with phobias and panic.

The evidence for the effectiveness of SSRIs as a treatment for phobias and panic is plentiful in the medical literature and many psychiatrists will prefer such treatments to psychological therapies, even when they are available and supported by evidence that they work. The prescribing of these drugs is, of course, reinforced by plentiful press reports of how effective they are for phobias and panic. What we also need to take into account, however, is the way in which the marketing of these drugs takes place.

Large drug companies have multi-million dollar budgets for marketing and, therefore, they have the resources to ensure that the use of these drugs is positively promoted in all forms of media. Although we have not quite reached the state of affairs in the USA, where the advertising of prescription-only medicines direct to the general public is widespread, it needs to be said that those who have phobias and panic may be somewhat misled by media accounts.

While I believe that the use of SSRIs for certain types of anxiety is justified, the downside of these medications needs to be clearly stated. One difficulty with the research on these drugs is that the vast majority of published studies lack long-term follow-up reports. Anyone reading such research papers will be struck by the short duration of these studies. The drugs concerned are often classed as effective because the studies show that there are benefits over a period of weeks or, at most, months. For many people, phobias and panic will often be lifelong disorders. Follow-up studies are needed to see what happens once the people studied stop taking the drug.

The discontinuation of these medications often leads to two substantial problems. The first is that the drugs generally work only for as long as people take them and when they stop taking them, they often revert to their previous condition. It is true that for some people with very severe phobias and panic, the drugs may provide them with a kick start on their road to recovery, but, more often than not, ending the drug treatment just puts them back at square one.

A major problem with these drugs is what drug companies like to refer to as 'the discontinuation syndrome' – that is, there are very significant problems with withdrawal. While it is true to say that some people may take an SSRI for many months then stop doing so and have few or no problems, many others find that they are as difficult to withdraw from as the Valium-like drugs, the benzodiazepines.

As I say, many people find that the drugs cause few or no side effects, other than some initial problems when they start taking them, but others experience side effects that can be more serious than their original problem. The commonest side effects that I see in my work are long-term weight gain and sexual problems. With regard to the former, weight gain often takes place gradually and, for some people, is impossible to reverse, even when they stop taking the medication. Sexual side effects are not so commonly reported, usually because people are embarrassed. Nevertheless, they are very common. Men often experience erectile problems and difficulties ejaculating and women may find that their ability to experience orgasm diminishes or disappears. In both men and women, SSRIs often lead to a reduction in sexual drive and interest.

My own view of these medications is that, for some, they might be beneficial, but there are two important issues that need to be addressed. The first is that the person prescribed such drugs should be very clearly and fully informed of their benefits and risks. The second is that, once the drug starts to be taken, its use should be very carefully monitored so that the person is not simply left with repeat prescriptions.

One condition for which SSRIs can be very effective is OCD. Then they are used in high doses and there is plentiful evidence that these drugs, either used on their own or, better still, together with an effective psychological treatment, can greatly improve what, at times, can be a severely handicapping problem. Such treatments for OCD probably need to be given indefinitely, however, as there is a great deal of evidence from clinical practice that, while it may be possible to reduce the dose, completely discontinuing it often leads to relapse.

Other antidepressants

While the guidelines on drug treatment for phobias and panic recommend SSRIs, many people are still prescribed other antidepressants. Sometimes this is because they have been taking the same drug for many years and GPs continue prescribing that rather than an SSRI. Some GPs and psychiatrists still have a preference for drugs other than SSRIs, particularly those in a group known as the tricyclic antidepressants.

These drugs include imipramine and amitriptyline and their use, based on research that is now 50 years old, is founded on the theory that they in some way block panic attacks. Tricyclic antidepressants probably work to overcome phobias and panic as a result of the sedative effect that they have.

Any potential user of such drugs needs to be aware that there are certainly short-term side effects, such as a dry mouth, blurred vision and constipation, which are often at troublesome levels. The long-term side effects, however, are much more serious. These may include enormous weight gain and effects on the heart and liver, which, in turn, increase the likelihood of life-threatening conditions.

Once more, dependence on these drugs is a problem and those who have been taking such medications for many years will need to follow withdrawal programmes similar to those advocated above for benzodiazepine tranquillizers.

Other medication

There have been a number of other kinds of medication suggested for the treatment of phobias and anxiety disorders. For example, the beta blocker group of drugs (primarily used in the treatment of high blood pressure) have been used to treat anxiety disorders for several decades. These drugs work by blocking physiological arousal and are sometimes helpful in the short term, but they clearly do not suit everyone. The side effects can be troublesome and range from tiredness, a sluggish feeling and slightly depressed mood to nightmares. Although one or two research studies have demonstrated that they are, in the short term, effective for anxiety disorders, the long-term results are not so good and, indeed, there is some evidence that people who use beta blocker drugs to combat anxiety in the long term may actually get worse rather than better.

Many people want to 'take something' for their anxiety, but do not want to take a prescription drug. It is therefore very common to hear of people who take St John's Wort (an effective treatment for mild to moderate depression, but probably not much help for anxiety disorders) and a range of natural remedies and homeopathic preparations. While I have no doubt that some people derive benefit from them because of a placebo effect (that is, they could be taking a sugar pill but their belief it will help them leads them to feel it has).

There is no research evidence for any of these alternative remedies having any place in the treatment of anxiety. My one additional note of caution is that, because natural remedies are unregulated in this country, you can never be completely sure what you are taking.

Psychotherapy

One of the difficulties regarding psychotherapy is its very definition. For many years, psychotherapy largely meant treatments based on the principles of psychoanalysis and, of course, Freud, Jung, Klein and others who were the main theoretical sources. In its original form, such therapy often took many years and sometimes involved people seeing their therapists up to five times a week.

The theory behind traditional psychotherapeutic treatments is that the symptoms are merely the product of an underlying conflict that often has its roots in childhood. I will not attempt to provide an overview of the theory of psychoanalytic treatments here, but suffice it to say that these supposed conflicts are very often linked to the psychoanalysts' ideas about childhood development.

One major difficulty associated with the psychoanalytical explanation of a variety of mental health problems is that they largely ignore any possible biological underpinnings of the problems. They also overlook the many and varied social factors that may be partly responsible for the cause and substantially maintain the difficulty in the longer term. Even when a basic cause in childhood or adolescence can be uncovered, another major difficulty is that the phobic problem may have been present for a number of years and by the time people visit a therapist the problems, in a sense, maintain themselves.

I accept that childhood experiences are important. Indeed, there is a body of research evidence that shows people with agoraphobia may have had traumatic separation experiences during crucial parts of their development. Many children who were separated from their parents during World War II as part of the evacuation programme went on to develop severe separation anxiety. Nevertheless, it is difficult to see how a psychotherapeutic process will deal with patterns of fear and avoidance.

Modern forms of psychotherapy come in various packages and are presented in different ways. For example, some therapists still maintain a close adherence to the traditional theories of psychoanalysis, while others say that they are not hugely influenced by the dim and distant figures of Freud and Jung. The problem that I have with such therapies is the lack of evidence. I could only recommend this form of treatment if it had been tested by a programme of rigorous research.

Self-help organizations

Although I devote much of this section to the organization of which I am the proud president and founding patron, No Panic, I have very sincere respect for other self-help organizations in the UK. I certainly believe that one of the central principles behind the self-help movement should be the more the merrier. Over 30 years or so, I have seen a number of organizations set up and prosper and others that have started with great enthusiasm and then entered terminal decline months or years afterwards.

I believe that we need some diversity in the types of self-help offered. It is clear that some organizations offer just what a particular individual needs and others do not. The main self-help organizations all advocate, as a central approach, self-help methods based on the best available evidence. Nevertheless, organizations also offer approaches that have not been tested for scientific studies, but are helpful to some, if not all.

Self-help groups offer different things to different people. All the main groups now have websites (some more user-friendly than others) and most of these provide helpful information about the nature of and treatments for fears and phobias. Some organizations offer a personal contact, which may be one of the most effective interventions for some people. Simply being in touch with someone who has a similar problem may lead to positive change. It is interesting how people – often with years of unsuccessful professional treatment up to this point – meet someone else who is in similar circumstances and they go on to encourage each other to achieve goals that they never realized in the course of their treatment.

Some organizations offer face-to-face contact, some group meetings, others telephone numbers, either between individuals or as a telephone conference group. With the advent of cheap and available web cameras and Skype technology, people can now see each other via the Internet and there is no charge. Members of some organizations that I know have set up instant message groups and there is, of course, a proliferation of contacts on Facebook, Bebo and other messaging media.

Do also see the Useful contacts section (p. 106) and browse the various websites to see what is on offer. To exemplify the work of these organizations, I will provide some information about No Panic.

No Panic

No Panic was set up for those with phobias, panic attacks, obsessive–compulsive disorders, general anxiety disorders and going through tranquillizer withdrawal.

It was started in late 1991 when Colin Hammond, who had had a recurrence of anxiety disorders, put an advert in the local paper telling people that he and his wife, Marion, were setting up a self-help group. The original idea was to run a group for people in Shropshire, where Colin and Marion lived, as there was no self-help organization for people with such disorders in their county.

Very quickly, they became inundated with telephone calls from across the West Midlands and, over a short period of time, No Panic became a national charity. At the time of writing this book, in the summer of 2009, the charity takes approximately 80,000 calls each year and the initial group of 4 volunteers has grown to nearly 100. There are now 3000 subscribing members and No Panic is also established in the Republic of Ireland with plans for similar groups in France and Spain.

No Panic offers a range of services for people who have phobias, panic attacks and the like and has an enormous resource of literature, audio and video cassettes and DVDs. Much of this material has been developed by No Panic members. The charity puts people in contact with others and offers a recovery programme delivered via the telephone. The recovery programme comes in different versions. The most popular is a telephone recovery group, which consists of an hour per week telephone course over a period of 14 weeks. The group networks people in a telephone conference format at cheap rate telephone times, usually in the evening, and there is no cost apart from the cost of the call. The 14-week programme takes people along the recovery pathway in graduated steps. The groups are led by people who have had anxiety disorders themselves and who have achieved some degree of recovery. These group coordinators have received training for the work that they do and No Panic ensures, as much as possible, that they have the highest ethical standards and are, of course, bound by confidentiality. The telephone recovery group is augmented by the use of a written manual, based on CBT principles, and members encourage each other in their endeavours to conquer their fears and phobias.

Other types of telephone contact involve group and individual mentoring programmes.

Like other self-help groups, No Panic is funded on a shoestring and derives its income from very modest member subscriptions and grants from the NHS and charities. Each year sees a new crisis regarding ensuring adequate funding. Given that No Panic and its sister charities provide such a service for, literally, hundreds of thousands of people, I find it incredible that the government gives so little in the way of support.

In addition, although many in the NHS recognize the importance of self-help organizations and 'talk the talk', loudly proclaiming the need for self-help organizations to work in close cooperation with NHS teams, when it comes to the implementation of this ideal there is usually a problem. There are some exceptions to this, some health professionals having gone out of their way to ensure that they work side by side with their self-help colleagues. Nevertheless, this level of cooperation needs to be extended. In my opinion, even when people are receiving plentiful professional help (which is still a rarity), the need for self-help in one form or another remains.

Part 2
THE SELF-HELP PROGRAMME

4

Introduction to the self-help programme

In the following chapters I will set out a complete self-help programme. It is aimed primarily at those with phobias, but may be of assistance to many of those with other anxiety problems. The programme consists of the following steps:

- defining your problem
- selecting your targets or goals
- deciding on and implementing your plan
- dealing with specific phobias
- managing panic and general anxiety
- evaluating your progress.

The following chapters each cover one of the above steps in turn, so when you have read them all you will have a clear picture of the whole of this programme of self-help treatment. Don't try to tackle them all in one go, however. I suggest that you read each chapter in your own time. When you have finished one, return to this chapter and then work your way through the rest of the chapters in order. Don't feel that you need to complete each chapter as quickly as possible – take your time. So, when, for example, you come to plan your treatment targets, make your list and then sleep on it. Return to your list the following day and ask yourself, 'Have I got that right? Do I need to add something more?' Equally, don't try to achieve the perfect plan. Try things out and, if they don't work out as you wished, take a step back and see how you can improve it.

Then, as I say to all those who come to me to embark on their treatment journeys: don't just think about it, do it!

5

Defining your problem

Although it may seem rather obvious, defining the precise nature of your problem is the first necessary step on your road to recovery.

It is essential to define exactly what the problem is in clear and unambiguous terms. For example, saying 'simply' that you are agoraphobic or you have panic attacks does not really describe the problem. It is rather like saying, 'My car is not running properly.' If you took your car to a garage you would provide the mechanic with more information than that – as much as possible, in fact – so that the problem could be diagnosed and sorted out.

If we take the example of agoraphobia, we can see just how much there is to the condition. The term generally indicates that a person is anxious about a number of particular situations. If this is you, to take this first step you need to find the answers to some basic questions. What is the nature of your anxiety? What physical symptoms do you experience? Does your anxiety include certain thoughts, such as 'I'm going to pass out', 'I'm going to collapse' or 'I must escape'? There may also be factors that make the anxiety better or worse. For example, using a walking stick may help if you have a fear of fainting or carrying a mobile telephone so that you can obtain help or knowing where the nearest exit is so you know you can get out – all these things will make you feel more secure. Likewise, carrying a bottle of water may help if you have a fear of choking. People with such fears often believe that they then have something to fall back on if the worst comes to the worst.

Alternatively, situations may be made worse by certain things. For example, the very bright lights in supermarkets may increase feelings of unreality, which may make some people feel like they might be going mad. Some women have much greater problems at certain times in their menstrual cycle, while others (men and women) may feel worse at night and so on.

All these factors mean that it is worth exploring your problem in some depth so you can see exactly what it is you are fighting, in clear detail. To continue with our example, someone might define their agoraphobic fear as follows.

- Fear of situations where there is no obvious escape, such as crowded buses, trains, theatres and supermarkets. This fear leads to an avoidance of such situations, which, in turn, restricts my ability to work, shop and socialize.
- The fear comprises thoughts connected with a loss of control (passing out, fainting, vomiting, collapsing, becoming incontinent). Although I know that these thoughts are irrational, exposure to my feared situations makes these thoughts feel overwhelming, to the point where I'm sure that these fears are about to become a reality.

The consistent avoidance of situations provoking such fears may lead to problems of lowered self-esteem and pessimism. People may compare themselves unfavourably with others and feel that the future has nothing to offer. In general, therefore, they may feel that they are failures. This then inhibits them from undertaking new hobbies, looking for a job and so on and eventually despair and depression may result.

It may be helpful to break the problem down in slightly different ways – by making a list of things that are causing you difficulty, for example.

- Try to identify exactly what it is that you are afraid of happening (collapsing, dying, fainting).
- Define the situations that cause the anxiety. When and where does it occur?
- Define how the avoidance of those situations leads to handicap. What effects does it have on you?

It is also worth attempting to identify what makes a situation better or worse. For example, a person with a fear of collapsing in the supermarket may find that holding their child's hand or even carrying a walking stick may give a helpful feeling of security.

These modifying factors are so important because they can be used in treatment. Thus, if there are three or four things that make a situation better, you should gradually practise doing without those things – but one at a time. Take small steps.

As I point out below, the plan for exposure to those situations that normally cause you difficulty should be carefully thought through. There should be an emphasis on gradually increasing exposure to them. Likewise, as mentioned, you should graduate your approach towards reducing your reliance on any modifying factors.

Conclusion

Defining your problem is the first step on your road to recovery. Make sure that you do the following:

- think about all the components that make up your problem
- identify those situations that cause you difficulty or you tend to avoid
- define the thoughts that trouble you
- identify all those factors that make the problem worse or better
- define how the problem upsets and/or interferes with your normal activities.

Once you have done this, you can begin to go on to the next stage, which is to select your treatment targets or goals.

6

Selecting your targets or goals

The very first question you should ask yourself is, 'What would I like to do that I can't do at present because of my problems?'

This is an important question and should be answered honestly. Be selfish: think about what you want; put to one side what you think others expect of you. You need to bear in mind that other people might, sometimes, want you to do things that you do not necessarily want to do for yourself.

Setting your targets should be a two-stage process. First, you must decide what goals (targets) you wish to achieve and then you should define each one in detail.

Developing your target areas

Having another look at your original list of problems should help you to see what targets you wish to aim for. For example, if your fear is of shopping centres and you enjoy shopping, your target might simply be to go shopping with a friend twice a week. If your fear is of underground trains and that is the quickest way to get to work, your target might be to travel to work using the tube. If your problem concerns panic, your target might be to face up to panicky feelings when they occur and use strategies designed to reduce or eliminate your symptoms.

If your problem stops you doing things that you enjoy, such as pursuing your hobbies or interests, you should begin by trying to develop targets that are enjoyable in their own right, but may involve exposure to situations that would normally cause you anxiety. Going to a football match or joining an evening class might be obvious examples.

Detailing your targets

As with problem statements, targets need to be specific. This is probably best illustrated by the following example.

Say that one of your targets is to 'Travel by underground train'. This phrase does not tell you very much about the precise behaviour you are aiming for and does not focus on the different aspects of the problem that must be tackled. A more suitable long-term (ultimate) target might be:

> To travel by underground from Arnos Grove Station to Piccadilly Circus, five times a week, in the rush hour. This journey will be undertaken alone, without the aid of the water bottle that I use to deal with the possibility that I might choke. During the journey I will practise observing fellow passengers, rather than distracting myself by listening to my iPod.

Obviously you may wish to develop your target behaviours in a more gradual way. Using the example above, instead your first target might be:

> To travel by underground train from Cockfosters to Southgate station (two stops, no long tunnels) after the rush hour finishes with a friend at least twice a week.

If your problem concerns shopping, your long-term (ultimate) target might be:

> To shop at least twice a week, for at least 90 minutes in Bluewater shopping centre on a busy day (a Friday evening or Saturday morning) and practise waiting in the longest queue in a noisy and brightly lit shop.

An intermediate target might be to spend 30 minutes in your local supermarket, twice a week, in quiet periods, accompanied by a friend or family member.

Ideally, each defined problem should have at least three goal (or target) statements attached to it. It does not matter how many targets you set, but it is worth considering how these may be broken down so that you can tackle them in stages. For example, you may choose to set targets to be achieved in the short term (within four weeks), medium term (within three months) and longer term (within six months to a year).

Write your targets down and display them in a place where you will see them frequently.

Conclusion

Drawing up a list of targets is the second step on your road to recovery. Make sure that you do the following:

- make a list of the things that you want to be able to do;

- be very specific about the detail of each target;
- make sure that the target reflects your problem statement;
- think about your targets in the short, medium and long term.

When you have made your list, show it to your spouse, partner or a trusted friend. You should do this so as to check whether or not there are additional targets you might wish to include. This also provides you with an opportunity to enlist support and practical help so that you can achieve your targets.

Keep your list of targets in a place where you will see them frequently.

7

Deciding on and implementing your plan

A central principle, reiterated throughout this book, is that exposure to the object or situation causing you anxiety is essential if you are to overcome your fears. Thus, the central element in your plan must be exposure to that which you fear. Other aspects of anxiety management and control are also important, however, such as paying attention to exercise, diet, time management, alcohol and sleep (see Chapter 9).

It is important that your plan is written down. Write down all the aspects of your plan you can think of and then consider them in the light of any constraints imposed by your normal routine or your life priorities. In my experience, if you are to overcome your phobia, your exposure plan needs to be a top priority in your life. If you cannot decide firmly that the plan is your number one priority, you will probably not succeed in overcoming your fears.

Drawing up your plan

First, if you experience phobic anxiety states, there is absolutely no doubt that you must plan to increase your exposure to your feared object or situation. I make no apologies for repeating this message over and over again. You must accept that recovery from the problem will involve you facing up to that which makes you afraid. The main principles of this approach are explored below.

Planning your exposure

In order to benefit from self-help, it is important to understand the details of the treatment method. Thus, the most helpful way to plan your treatment is to consider how exposure can be used most effectively to help you overcome your difficulties. In describing the possible approaches, I have drawn on the results of a considerable amount of research that has been carried out worldwide and my own clinical experience.

The use of exposure in your imagination and real life

As we saw in Chapter 3, the early treatment methods of the 1950s and 1960s relied on people training their imagination. Simply, people were taught to imagine their feared situation and then how to relax while they thought about it.

Over the years, exposure simply in people's imagination became redundant and therapists emphasized the need for people to face up to their fears in real life. Now, however, there is ample evidence that using your imagination can, in fact, be very helpful in the early stages of treatment.

What you need to do is quite simple. Try to imagine yourself in the situation or facing the object you fear while at the same time seeing yourself calmly staying there and coping with that situation. This can be a very helpful way to prepare yourself for the real thing.

Most people with phobias will try to push any thoughts about their phobic object from their mind. You should really try to do the opposite. Try thinking about the situation or object for as long as possible, but at least ten minutes at a time.

How often should I expose myself to the phobic object or situation and for how long?

Research shows very clearly that long sessions of exposure are much more effective than short ones. That is because, put simply, you need to allow yourself time to calm down.

You will feel like you are beginning to calm down after a few minutes, but to have a lasting effect on reducing your anxiety often takes much longer. So, the longer you can stay in the situation the better, because your body can only keep up high levels of adrenaline output for relatively brief periods. In addition, the longer your exposure continues, the more you will realize that what you fear will happen won't.

Ideally, then, exposure sessions should last two hours. Although this may sound like a tall order, there is a great deal of evidence to show that this amount of time is much more effective than shorter periods of 30 minutes or so. Regular practice is important, too.

The simple rule of thumb is that, if at all possible, you should face your fears on a daily basis. My experience is that doing as much as you possibly can will always be more helpful than being conservative. I believe that there is very little risk from frequent sessions and that, although many people anticipate that they may 'overdo it', it is unlikely.

How gradual should my exposure be?

Some people can progress very quickly to facing their most feared object or situation; others may take a little longer. People are different! Some can very quickly graduate to doing the worst thing that they can imagine (for example, travelling on a crowded underground train in the rush hour), while others need to approach their fears very gradually.

Research does not really reveal any conclusive evidence either way. A simple rule of thumb is to do what is difficult, but just about manageable.

Do I need to experience anxiety during exposure sessions?

Although most people dread exposure treatment and anticipate that they will have very high levels of anxiety, the amount they experience when they actually confront their feared situation or object is very variable. Indeed, a significant minority of people experience very little anxiety when they eventually face up to a situation that they may have avoided for many years.

The simple answer is that it does not seem to matter how much anxiety you experience during an exposure session, provided you continue to have exposure sessions, as often and for as long as you can.

Going it alone versus working with others

Some research shows that group treatment sessions can be very effective in overcoming phobias and panic in some individuals. It appears that facing your fears with others often provides additional confidence, motivation and reinforcement. Many of the treatment programmes I have run in hospital outpatient settings have involved group approaches. The camaraderie that develops is very positive and several people develop enduring friendships with their fellow phobics. Group treatment is not for everybody, though, and some people simply wish to do it on their own.

If you are a member of a self-help group, you may be offered a group approach. No Panic, for example, uses a telephone conference system, whereby people 'meet' once a week on the telephone via a conference call system. The purposes of such groups are to set each other targets and provide encouragement and support. Again, some people find it very helpful, but others would rather go it alone.

Remember that, although you should accept as much practical help as possible from others, your ultimate goal is to be able to face your phobic situations or objects alone. You should, therefore, always be aware that having someone with you should be seen as an intermediate step on the way. Excessive dependence on others may eventually be detrimental.

Do I need a professional therapist?

The straightforward answer to this question is generally 'No'. Provided that you can follow the central principle of facing your fears and those around you are supportive, following a plan of increasing exposure may be as good as receiving help from a professional therapist. Professional therapists can provide an objective assessment of your problem, however, and the encouragement you need to face the situation or object.

As mentioned earlier, many years ago, therapists (myself included) spent literally hundreds of hours every year with people, helping them to face their feared situations. We accompanied them so as to coax and encourage them to face up to their fears. Although there were some excellent results from this approach, it also had its drawbacks. Apart from the obvious issues of cost, people could become overly reliant on their therapists and all that time may merely have been a way of putting off the inevitable moment when people had to face their fears alone.

As a rule of thumb, I would say that if therapist-aided exposure is indicated, this should be to introduce you to the situation, after which the therapist should fade into the background. Unless there are exceptional reasons, six sessions of therapist assistance should be the maximum.

Having a cotherapist

Facing any problem generally proves more successful if you have the help and encouragement of those around you. It therefore makes sense to enlist the aid of a cotherapist. Your cotherapist, however, needs to know what to do and when to do it.

Most people with phobias and panic receive considerable help from others, but, unless it is carefully thought through, such help can, at times, be counterproductive. For example, the spouse or partner of someone with agoraphobia may take on a number of the responsibilities that that person would normally undertake for him- or herself. In the end, such a shift in responsibilities may be detrimental and promote an increased dependency on others. The partner may also get drawn into giving endless and meaningless reassurance and, eventually, seeking that reassurance may become the main point of any interaction. The partner may also become an extra source of security, being with the person day and night and accompanying him or her whenever a feared situation must be faced.

If you choose to enlist the help of a cotherapist, he or she should recognize that previous behaviour might have been counterproductive. It is not always easy to break old habits, so the treatment plan may have to involve the cotherapist gradually changing his or her behaviour as well. Cotherapists should, therefore, read books such as this one thoroughly and be totally involved with the planning of the programme. That is not to say they should take over the running of the programme as, if they did, it would just reinforce their partner's dependency.

The role of your cotherapist, then, is to provide encouragement and assistance, help you face up to your feared and avoided situations or objects and, at the same time, provide ongoing support and encouragement. This, like many other things, is easier said than done. There will, of course, be pitfalls. If, however, you and your cotherapist review progress objectively, perhaps using the diaries described below, many of these pitfalls may be avoided.

Keeping a diary

There are numerous ways in which you can keep a diary, but three examples are provided below.

The first is a general diary (see Table 1) wherein day-to-day activities and ratings as to the level of your anxiety and mood are noted. Recording such information over a period of time will help you to see the relationships between what you do and how you feel. The 'Comments' section on the far right can be used to summarize your overall view of the day.

Table 1 Example of a general diary

Date	Main events of the day	High/low anxiety points*	Mood ratings**	Comments

Notes
* Score anxiety on a scale from 0 to 8, where 0 = no anxiety and 8 = worst anxiety possible.
**Score depression on a scale from 0 to 8, where 0 = no problems and 8 = worst depression possible.

The second type of diary – an exposure diary – is specific to exposure tasks and is used to record the length of your sessions and your anxiety ratings (see Table 2).

You should record your anxiety ratings before, during and after a session. It is also important to note whether or not a cotherapist has been present, then plan your next task.

This simple format can be modified and extra columns added as required.

Table 2 Example of an exposure diary

Date	Exposure situation	Length of session	Anxiety ratings*	Cotherapist present?	Next task planned

Note
* Score anxiety on a scale from 0 to 8, where 0 = no anxiety and 8 = worst possible anxiety.

The thoughts diary (see Table 3) can be particularly valuable for those who experience panic attacks as it helps you to identify various patterns of negative and catastrophic thoughts.

This is an important process that acts as a first step in managing the thoughts associated with panic attacks. Various strategies that you can adopt are described in the next chapter.

Table 3 Example of a thoughts diary

Date	Situation	Triggers	Thoughts	Consequences

Overall, diaries of how you feel, what you do and how successful you are provide perhaps the best way to evaluate your progress. You should keep your original list of problems and targets and use the diaries as a way of determining how close you are to achieving the targets you have set for yourself.

It may well be that, after a while, your targets need to be revised and, indeed, it may become clear as you go on that your view of your problem changes. In this case, you will need to revise your original definition. This often happens when you have avoided something for a long time and it is not until you begin to face it that you start to see things in a different light.

8

Dealing with specific phobias

The same rules of exposure apply to managing specific phobias as to the more complex phobias, such as agoraphobia. Gradual exposure to the feared situation or object is the central approach (see p. 74).

Each type of phobia may call for some additional strategies to deal with problems specific to that phobia. For example, in the case of a vomiting phobia, secondary problems, such as checking behaviours or an obsession with sell-by dates and the state of food in the fridge, would need to be dealt with.

One approach would be to let someone else take responsibility for cooking as he or she might also have a more relaxed attitude to sell-by dates. Giving up control for someone with such a phobia is a real step forward.

Similarly, the phobic person may have avoided drinking alcohol. In such a case, I would advise drinking alcohol on a regular basis. Note that this is contrary to my general advice to people with phobias!

Vomiting phobias often involve people seeking reassurance so a ban on such behaviour may be part of a treatment plan for such a person.

Finally, this phobia is one that lends itself very well to using the imagination to aid recovery. If as a way of increasing exposure to the phobic situation, the person imagines him- or herself being sick on a very regular basis, this can be a very potent part of his or her treatment strategy.

To take another example, if someone has a fear of heights, simply trying to conquer taller and taller buildings will probably not be sufficient. The plan should involve a wide range of situations that involve facing this fear – looking out through a window, standing on a balcony, driving across a road bridge, crossing a bridge over water on foot, sitting on a bench at the top of a cliff and so on.

Such exposure to heights should perhaps be undertaken more frequently than exposure to other phobic situations. This is important because, as well as the normal physical sensations of fear, the person will also need to get used to the dizziness and the sense of falling. In this respect, having someone to accompany the person as he or she gains confidence is important, as long as the person doesn't hang on to his or her arms!

With this fear it is also a good idea to use films and computer programs that feature heights as a means of increasing exposure to them. In general, such strategies are often helpful in preparing the individual concerned for the real thing.

I have used simulation programs and so on to help treat other phobias. For example, in the case of people with a flying phobia who fear turbulence, the use of a flight simulator at an aircraft museum has been invaluable.

Social phobias present a very wide range of challenges. Not only do social situations have their particular difficulties but also the particular aspects of each person's fear need to be carefully considered. In the example of someone who fears blushing, one might suggest a ban on make-up used to camouflage the blushing skin. It could also be suggested that he or she observes others to see them coping with similar problems.

Treatment approaches need to be specifically tailored to both the phobia in question and the individual circumstances. It may be helpful to describe the treatment of a patient with a bird phobia to illustrate, in a detailed way, how self-help treatments can work.

Liz

Liz had a phobia of pigeons for as long as she could remember. She recalled several occasions as a child when her phobia prevented her from going on school journeys and she remembers being unable to go to the National Gallery in London because it is on one side of Trafalgar Square where there are thousands of pigeons.

Birds other than pigeons also made her feel uncomfortable, but it was pigeons in particular that caused her to feel very panicky and she sometimes had nightmares about them flying into her face. She remembers that she went to see the Hitchcock movie *The Birds* and had to leave after about 15 minutes. On some occasions she came across groups of pigeons and, in her words, became 'hysterical'.

When Liz left school she did not need to visit places with pigeons as she worked in a quiet suburban office. Her problem came to the fore, though, when she started to go out with a young man who was an avid football fan.

She accompanied him to a match for the first time and was horrified to find flocks of pigeons near the entrance to the ground. Although she managed to keep herself under control, she found that her whole experience of the match was overwhelmed by her vision of the flocks of pigeons that she had encountered before the match. She also anticipated the terror that she would experience when she had to go through the entrance again when the match ended.

She did not tell her boyfriend about her fear and he was therefore mystified as to why she was so withdrawn during the match.

The following week her boyfriend suggested that they went to London to see a film and Liz happily agreed. They arrived early, however, and, to her horror, he suggested that they went to the National Gallery to pass the time. At this point she broke down and told him about her phobia. Shortly afterwards, she decided to seek treatment.

Following a thorough assessment, the therapist decided that Liz was a suitable candidate for self-treatment – that she should plan and implement her own exposure programme. After some considerable discussion, Liz and her therapist agreed that she should do a number of things to prepare herself for facing pigeons in real life. Liz realized that, if she was to overcome her fear, she would eventually need to make a trip to Trafalgar Square. The very thought of doing so filled her with horror; even talking about it made her heart beat faster and she broke into a sweat.

Liz began by setting herself a number of exercises directed towards helping her to begin the process of exposure to her feared object. First, she joined the Royal Society for the Protection of Birds (RSPB) and, along with her subscription, came a number of leaflets and a magazine filled with pictures. She then managed to obtain some copies of videos of birds and, after visiting several toy shops, she found a cardboard cut-out of a pigeon that she suspended over her bed. In the course of the next three weeks, she looked at the pictures and watched the videos and, every morning, she woke up to see the cardboard pigeon swinging from her bedroom ceiling.

The next step was to find pigeons that she could observe from a distance. She found that pigeons tended to congregate at her local shopping centre. She thus positioned herself a little distance away from them and made herself watch the pigeons for 20 to 25 minutes at a time.

Following these exercises, her next exposure task was to visit the Snowdon Aviary at London Zoo. Although, coincidentally, she saw a few pigeons there from a distance, her main task in going there was to expose herself to other birds that, prior to her treatment, had made her feel uncomfortable. She now felt, however, that she could begin to face up to the birds in the aviary as a way of preparing herself for closer contact with pigeons.

After meeting with her therapist again to review progress, it was agreed that Liz should try to imagine herself in Trafalgar Square with a group of pigeons and keep this image in her mind for as long as possible. The therapist instructed her to imagine herself coping with the experience and throwing some breadcrumbs for the birds. At the same time, she agreed to keep the other exposure exercises going. Although she found that the self-treatment exercises consumed a great deal of her time, Liz had begun to feel better about facing pigeons and her trips to the shopping centre evoked much less anxiety than they would have done previously.

Some six weeks after her first assessment, and following only two brief sessions with the therapist, Liz spontaneously decided that she should enlist the help of her boyfriend and take a trip to Charing Cross Station, then walk as close as she could to Trafalgar Square to observe the flocks of pigeons there from a distance. She managed to stand on the other side of the road, away from the main square. She spent half an hour there in the company of her boyfriend and, during that period of time, her anxiety level dropped from her initial high rating of 7 to 4 (out of a maximum of 8). (Liz's therapist had instructed her on the use of the anxiety rating scale shown on p. 79).

After her visit, Liz was very pleased with her progress and telephoned her therapist. The therapist suggested that Liz should repeat the exercise and, this time, try to make it to the edge of the square itself. She did this successfully and surprised herself by feeling calm enough after 15 minutes to take a few tentative steps on her own into Trafalgar Square. At that point a pigeon flew very close to her head and she panicked. Nevertheless, having previously discussed the possibility of an incident such as this with her therapist, she took a few minutes to compose herself and set off once more into the square.

After another phone call to her therapist, Liz repeated the exposure exercise and, after four more trips to Trafalgar Square, found that she was able to take the final step of feeding the pigeons that gathered at her feet.

Six months after her treatment had finished, Liz visited her therapist for a review. Liz agreed that she was now able to go about her daily life without being preoccupied with birds. She proudly reported that she had made three trips to the National Gallery with her boyfriend. She was still slightly anxious when she saw a pigeon or a group of pigeons in the street, but she said that she felt she was over her problem.

Liz's story illustrates the step-by-step approach to exposure and shows how a problem can be broken down into difficult, but manageable, steps. In Liz's case, her therapist really only needed to see her for one long session of assessment, taking about an hour and a half. Her subsequent therapy, including telephone conversations, required approximately another hour and a half.

9

Managing panic and general anxiety

Managing panic

Panic management essentially comprises three central approaches. The first, and perhaps the most important, is to maintain exposure. That means you should prevent yourself from 'escaping' from the situation, which brings us to the other two main elements of panic management. These are dealing with hyperventilation and, finally, dealing with catastrophic thoughts.

Hyperventilation

When we become anxious, our body's reaction is to prepare for 'fight or flight'. One element of this reaction is that we breathe more rapidly to provide the body with the additional oxygen it requires. In a state of anxiety and panic, however, the increase in our breathing is not required to help us to fight or flee from our foe! We are, in effect, breathing in excess of what our body actually needs.

Over time such hyperventilation (sometimes also called over-breathing) will lead to an imbalance in body chemistry. That is because there will be a reduction in carbon dioxide levels, which, in turn, changes the acid to alkali balance of the blood. The consequences of these changes in body chemistry are many and various, including sensations such as pins and needles, feeling light-headed, yawning or sighing and, in extreme cases, muscle spasms. Hyperventilating for extended periods of time also causes fatigue and sleepiness.

For those who have panic attacks, the symptoms produced by hyperventilation are frightening in themselves and, taken with other symptoms of anxiety, such as a rapid heart rate, they may feel that they are just about to have a stroke or a heart attack. As a result, the body produces more adrenaline, which, in turn, makes matters worse by feeding into a downward spiral of anxiety.

There is considerable evidence to show that teaching people to breathe more appropriately can be very effective in helping to reduce hyperventilation. The difficulty for some people is that panic develops so abruptly they do not realize that they are doing it.

Dealing with hyperventilation

Although people are taking in more air, hyperventilation usually leads to the breathing being shallow, restricted to the upper part of the chest, and rapid.

Simple breathing exercises, consisting of taking slow, but not too deep, breaths can be extremely helpful. Ensuring that your breathing comes from the diaphragm, rather than from the top of your chest, is very important. You can check that you are achieving this by placing your hand on your abdomen, slightly below your ribcage. Your tummy should move in and out to ensure that as much of the chest as possible is used.

Generally speaking, people who hyperventilate can reverse the pattern of overbreathing by practising the slow diaphragmatic breathing described above once or twice a day, combining this, if possible, with a period of physical relaxation. They should also try to undertake physical exercise (such as running, cycling, swimming, walking) as a regular part of their daily programme (see p. 89).

Some people who hyperventilate benefit from a medical device that is primarily used to lower blood pressure, but others find that there is less of an improvement. One example of such a device is called RESPeRATE. It consists of a chest lead with a sensor that you adjust to suit you, a headset and a small control box. The control box analyses your breathing and creates a melody, played through the headset, to guide your breathing. This works because research has established that learning to pace your breathing can relax the muscles around your blood vessels, leading to a reduction in blood pressure.

One benefit of this device for people with anxiety disorders who hyperventilate is that they can learn to pace their breathing so they breathe gently and diaphragmatically at a slow rate, which is calming and relaxing. People who use the machine to treat their high blood pressure often report how relaxed they feel after a treatment session.

I recommend that you don't expect immediate results. It may take six weeks before you feel any beneficial effects. Many people, though, report that their symptoms started to improve after a few days. After the initial six weeks, if you are feeling improvements, continue to use the device at least three times a week on an indefinite basis. Although such a machine does not come free, in my opinion, for those with very difficult to treat hyperventilation, it is a worthwhile investment.

There are some physiotherapists who specialize in teaching breath control, but, unfortunately, they are few and far between. In many areas, no such service is offered on the NHS. Indeed, the service is generally hard to find in the independent sector. If this is the situation where you live, you could try yoga or relaxation classes or a relaxation CD. See also Managing general anxiety, p. 88.

What to do in the case of acute panic

If possible, try to find somewhere quiet to either sit or lie down and endeavour to take slow breaths, breathing slowly from the diaphragm. It is helpful to loosen your clothing and relax your posture to make this easier. Although this can be very difficult, try to concentrate on relaxing your muscles and, at the same time, remember that panic can do no real harm.

One very rapid and effective way to deal with the hyperventilation associated with panic is the old tried and tested method of rebreathing exhaled air. Exhaled air contains more carbon dioxide than the air around us, so rebreathing it replenishes the carbon dioxide in your body, thus reversing the chemical changes that follow from hyperventilation, as described above.

You can rebreath exhaled air by breathing in and out of a paper bag, the top gathered in one hand and placed over your mouth. If this is not possible, a simple alternative is to cup your hands over your nose and mouth and rebreathe your exhaled air in that way. Doing this for two or three minutes is generally enough to restore the correct chemical balance in the body.

If you are in the company of someone who is hyperventilating, one of the key principles in managing the problem is to remain calm yourself. It is important to remember that hyperventilation, though it can look quite dramatic, is usually self-limiting and very rarely has any serious medical consequences. Very occasionally it can lead to muscular spasm, but this in itself is also harmless and self-limiting. It is the body's way of stopping overbreathing until the chemical balance is restored. Stay with the person and try to ensure that he or she remains still. Try to help the person relax and emphasize the need to breathe slowly and from the diaphragm. Use the paper bag or cupped hands techniques described above so that the person can rebreathe his or her expired air.

Dealing with catastrophic thoughts

If you keep a record of your panic attacks, perhaps using a diary (see p. 79), you will find that the thoughts accompanying such attacks will be much the same each time. For most people, the central theme tends to be the fear of some sort of loss of control. For example, you may fear that you will faint, have a stroke or a heart attack, vomit, go mad or die.

One of the most important ways to deal with such catastrophic thoughts is to examine the evidence. For example, you may have panicked on numerous occasions but when did this lead to anything other than anxiety about what could happen? Did you have a heart attack? Did you faint?

There is a range of strategies that might assist in keeping your thinking balanced. One such method is to write down a list of pros and cons – that is, points for and against the catastrophic outcome occurring. Then you can make up some small cards to carry in your wallet or purse to read if you feel panicky.

I often see people who can easily understand that their fears are very irrational, but, when they are faced with their feared situation and panic develops, the ability to think rationally disappears. One strategy that sometimes works is to record some rational, coping statements on a media player and listen to them in, for example, a crowded train carriage where the panic attacks occur.

Another strategy for dealing with catastrophic thoughts is to deliberately bring the thoughts on. It may sound very perverse, but give it a try – it often works. Psychologists and psychiatrists call this method paradoxical intention. Research by anxiety disorder experts has shown that facing these thoughts gives people a feeling that they are in control, rather than the thoughts controlling them, and so they feel much more able to tackle such patterns of thoughts than they did previously.

Remember that panic is harmless and self-limiting and other people are usually completely unaware that anything is happening. Also, in the longer term, escaping will only make the panic worse. What you should attempt to do is stay in the situation, however hard that seems, breathe slowly and repeat to yourself that nothing will happen. Recall your past experiences – although you may have thought that a heart attack or stroke was imminent, it has never happened. Remind yourself, too, that the body can only pump out adrenaline for brief periods of time and your symptoms are likely to be due to the high levels of adrenaline rather than anything more sinister.

Managing general anxiety

For those with phobias and panic, there are five important areas that are worth concentrating on in attempts to reduce the general level of anxiety. These are:

- exercise

- relaxation
- alcohol
- diet
- time management.

Exercise

There is plentiful evidence to suggest that regular and sensible exercise reduces the risk of a very wide range of diseases and people who exercise regularly report a reduction in their levels of anxiety, tension and depression. Indeed, NICE recommends regular aerobic exercise as a first-line treatment for mild to moderate depression.

The message regarding exercise is one that all those who experience anxiety should take on board. It is worth emphasizing, too, that age is certainly no barrier to using exercise as a strategy for reducing anxiety and tension. People who have serious health problems should exercise reasonably, in keeping with their underlying condition, however.

Below are some important rules regarding the most effective ways to exercise, but all forms of exercise, from gardening or playing golf to walking, are to be encouraged. For those with absolutely no background in any moderate to strenuous exercise, you simply need to begin by increasing your level of activity in general terms, whether this be by walking an extra ten minutes each day, hitting a few golf balls or even doing more housework. What is important is that you start.

Research evidence has now accumulated over many years and suggests very strongly that, for exercise to be effective in making us less susceptible to physical illnesses and to improve our mood and reduce tension, it needs to be at a reasonable level of intensity and repeated at least five times each week.

What is reasonable intensity?

The answer is exercise that maintains 70 to 80 per cent of your maximum heart rate.

How do I calculate my maximum heart rate?

The answer is simple. Maximum heart rate is calculated as 220 minus your age. Therefore, for a 20-year-old, the maximum heart rate is 200 and 70 to 80 per cent of his or her maximum heart rate is therefore 140 to 160 beats per minute.

One of the simplest ways to determine whether or not you are exercising strenuously enough is the talking test. If you are exercising at around 70 to 75 per cent of your maximum heart rate, you should be able to hold a conversation, but somewhat out of breath and perspiring.

Prior to embarking on any exercise, and particularly if you have any health problems, you should consult your GP. If you are over 40 years of age and have not exercised for a number of years (even if you feel that you are in good health) you should still consult your GP and tell him or her that you intend to begin a programme of exercise. If you have not seen your GP in recent times, he or she will probably want to check your blood pressure and may carry out a simple examination, which may include simple blood tests to check for common problems such as anaemia.

Obviously, even if your GP gives you the all clear, if you have not exercised for a long time you cannot simply go straight into a programme of five-times-a-week exercise that gets your heart beating at 70 to 75 per cent of its maximum. Your approach needs to be one of building up to this gradually.

You might start by simply walking and jogging for 20 minutes at a time, 3 times a week, gradually building up your stamina. Increasing your exercise by 10 per cent per week, you will soon build up a reasonable pattern of exercise. Your aim should be to exercise 5 times per week for 30 minutes each time.

To achieve this, you need to engage in activities such as running, rowing, cycling, swimming or using a cross-trainer at a gym. Ideally you should mix these different activities so that you exercise different parts of your body. Swimming is great for increasing suppleness and use of the cross-trainer will exercise your arms and legs. Note that you will not attain the required improvement to your heart rate by going for a long walk in the country, playing golf or pushing a shopping trolley around the supermarket.

Exercising on your own is difficult, particularly in the dark winter months. Exercising with a friend will keep you motivated. Leisure centres and gyms often have excellent facilities and employ qualified fitness instructors who will usually be able to offer you assistance with an exercise plan. There is some cost involved, but this is a worthwhile investment in your health. You could try group classes, too, such as spinning, which uses static cycles, or aerobics classes.

The Exercise on Prescription Programme

The majority of those with anxiety and panic will probably be eligible for the 'Exercise on Prescription Programme'. This scheme generally operates for people over 15 who have some of the risk factors associated with coronary heart disease. These risk factors include being a smoker, having high cholesterol, a family history of heart disease, high blood pressure, a stressful lifestyle or being overweight.

The programme, which is funded by the government, can also be offered to people to improve mobility, help with the control of diabetes and, most relevant to readers of this book, assist with the treatment of depression.

To find out if you qualify for this programme, simply ask your GP to refer you. If you are eligible, he or she will complete a prescription card and refer you to the nearest health and fitness adviser at a local leisure centre. This will be followed by a consultation with him or her that will involve an explanation of the scheme, a talk about relevant medical conditions and an assessment of your current physical activity levels. This initial consultation is then followed by a fitness assessment, with measurements of height, weight, body fat composition and exercise tolerance.

Once you have started your exercise programme, you will be offered support and guidance for 12 weeks. This 12 weeks may involve a wide range of types of exercise to not only improve your ability to exercise at 70 to 75 per cent of your maximum heart rate but also work on your general fitness, including building up strength in your abdomen, legs and upper body.

In 2007, the Department of Health published a very positive evaluation of the programme. The results show quite clearly that any costs involved are amply returned by increases in the health of the population.

In my opinion, anyone with a significant anxiety problem who is registered with a GP should be eligible for this scheme.

How does exercise assist someone who has a phobia state but is not generally anxious?

Even if your phobia is very specific and confined to particular social situations, objects or animals, engaging in regular physical exercise will help as it lowers the level of adrenaline in your body, thus making you less susceptible to anxiety. When you are attempting to face your fears, it is often very helpful to exercise before you do so. The following case study is just one example of this.

Alex
Alex had a particular phobia of attending meetings at work when they were held in rooms that he felt it was difficult to get out of. In all other ways, Alex is a very normal young man who describes himself as 'relaxed in personality and outlook'. Indeed, when I first met Alex, he was – like many people with a specific social anxiety – very relaxed and laid back.

At our first interview, Alex radiated charm and confidence and he had excellent social skills. As the interview progressed, however, he told me about his fear of meetings at work and his specific concern that he might become anxious, his workmates might notice this and they would think badly of him. He was also preoccupied with the fear that, if he became anxious at such a meeting, he might lose control, but he was unable to tell me how he would lose control. When we discussed his fears further, he told me: 'I realize that if my workmates thought I was anxious, nothing would happen. Indeed, I know one of them had panic attacks several years ago that were so bad he needed to take three weeks off work. Nevertheless, part of my brain tells me, despite my rational view of everything, that I will become overwhelmed by anxiety and lose control. I think if that happened it would be a total disaster.'

When we considered his problem in more depth, it became clear that one of the major components of Alex's anxiety was his anticipation that there would be problems. When a meeting was fixed for, say, a Friday, by Tuesday he would already be thinking about ways that he might excuse himself from attending or, if this was not possible, he would become increasingly preoccupied by a catastrophe that he believed lay ahead.

When I asked Alex to tell me more about this pattern of anticipation, he told me that some of his anticipation was along the lines of catastrophic thinking – that is, he imagined all the worst possible outcomes.

Another part of his pattern of anticipation was the physical tension he experienced, his palpitations and butterflies.

We developed some plans to help Alex deal with his anxiety, which included making a pact with himself to never avoid such situations and always to face them. We also developed strategies for thinking in a different way about his fears of being humiliated and losing control. The major strategy we employed, however, was physical exercise.

Alex was 26 years old and had stopped exercising when he went to university at 18. Over the past few years he had been too busy to exercise and become rather unfit. I therefore persuaded him to join a gym and start some of his old activities, which included swimming and kick-boxing. He also started to run on the treadmill, although it was not his preferred activity.

After six weeks or so of gradually increasing the amount of physical exercise he did, Alex reported sleeping better and was very pleased that he had lost some of his abdominal fat and 3 kg in weight.

He identified the mornings of days when he had meetings scheduled as times when exercise could be used to good effect as he noted that, after a reasonable workout at the gym, he felt relaxed for several hours afterwards and that, during and after exercise, worries tended to clear from his mind.

So, Alex put into operation a plan that included strategies for dealing with his thoughts. Before he went to work on a meeting day, he exercised for 45 minutes. This involved getting up earlier than usual and going for a run, as the leisure centre was not conveniently located in relation to his house.

Over a period of four to five months, Alex became much more effective at dealing with his anxiety regarding meetings and, although by the end of treatment, they still caused him some anxiety, he realized that it was tolerable. He also told me, without prompting, that he now believed it was quite normal to have some anxiety when dealing with the issues that were part of his job. Also that, over time, he had begun to realize others demonstrated anxiety in these situations, too.

Part of Alex's treatment involved observing others for signs of anxiety and, during the time that I knew him, Alex attended a conference where he listened to a speaker whom he much admired. He noticed that, at the beginning of her presentation, her voice faltered slightly and her hands had a slight tremor. He also noticed that these signs of anxiety disappeared and, at the end of her presentation, he joined in with others in the audience and gave her a standing ovation. He, thus, learned a very valuable lesson – that anxiety can coexist with success.

Returning to exercise, by the time Alex's treatment with me had been completed, he had joined a martial arts club and was a regular attender at the local gym. He told me that one additional benefit of his exercise programme was that it gave him a better work–life balance and he could not now envisage his life without exercise!

I am too busy to exercise

I am sure that every health professional who has advocated exercise as a remedy for anything at all has heard this plaintive cry. My simple response to this is that the week consists of 168 hours and exercising 5 times a week for 30 minutes, with some additional time for travelling there and back, getting changed and showering afterwards, will take something in the order of 7 to 8 hours. That is two and a half hours of exercise and four and a half hours or so of travel and preparation. That still leaves 160 hours in the week.

My simple view is that if you can't give up something in the order of 5 per cent of your overall time to one of the most valuable life activities, then there is surely something wrong with your life. Work out how many hours you spend in front of the TV, channel hopping, how long you spend, either at work or at home, staring into space or surfing the Internet.

I remember the words of famous football manager Bill Shankly when he was asked whether football was a matter of life or death. His answer was, 'No, it's more important than that.' I think in some ways this humorous riposte, for those with anxiety disorders, has a very serious message. Exercise may be of not only considerable assistance in helping you overcome your fears, phobias or panic but also the difference between health and illness.

There are, of course, some notes of caution – the principal one being that people who have very high levels of stress and find that exercise produces relief can sometimes find themselves becoming addicted to exercise itself. I frequently come across cases of people who exercise to the point of obsession, their physical health, ironically, becoming grossly impaired. Such an obsession is, of course, a problem in its own right. Despite this risk, exercise is probably the most important of all the stress management strategies and can lead to a great improvement in people's quality of life. For lots of information about sport and exercise, visit the website <www.sportengland.org>.

Relaxation

Although relaxation is not used directly as a treatment for either phobias or panic attacks, it can often be helpful in reducing the general level of physical arousal and body tension. The instructions that follow give you an introduction if you want to have a try. Otherwise, there are various relaxation exercises available on CDs or in other forms.

Relaxation training

Relaxation training is a helpful way to reduce the consequences of anxiety and panic.

While there are many ways to achieve relaxation, most focus on a systematic tensing and relaxing of the muscles in the body. This has two benefits. First, it helps you to differentiate between states of tension and relaxation and, importantly, recognize when your level of muscle tension is increasing. Second, there is considerable evidence to suggest that systematic tensing and relaxing exercises eventually lead to a state of overall muscle relaxation and a consequent feeling of well-being.

The following instructions are straightforward. It may be helpful to read and inwardly digest them, then make a recording that you can follow. If you do this, however, remember to leave a ten-second gap between each phase. This may be as effective as any commercially available recording and is certainly worth trying as, unlike them, it is free!

First of all, identify a time in the day when you have 30 minutes to devote to this task. Find a quiet room, take the phone off the hook and wear loose, comfortable clothing. The exercise can be carried out in a comfortable chair or lying down and you should experiment with different situations and times of the day to identify what the optimum conditions are for you.

Before doing the exercises, it is important to remember that, when tensing your muscles, this should be done to a moderate extent. If you tense them too hard, you will defeat the object of the exercise. A simple guide is that it should lead to no more than a sensation of tension or 'pulling'; if you experience pain, you're trying too hard. Further, when you release the tension, you should feel it go immediately.

Get in position and begin with your right hand. Clench your fist so that your knuckles are white. Hold for five seconds then release immediately.

Pause, wait ten seconds, then repeat.

Tense your right forearm, closing your fist and tensing the muscles of your forearm. Remember, not too hard. Hold for five seconds then release immediately.

Pause, wait ten seconds, then repeat.

Tense your right biceps, clenching your fist and bending your arm so it forms a 90-degree angle. Concentrate on making your biceps bulge as much as possible. Hold for five seconds then release immediately.

Pause, wait ten seconds, then repeat.

Repeat these actions with the left hand, forearm and biceps, remembering to do each exercise twice, hold for five seconds, then release immediately.

Next, move to your head and neck. Tense your eye muscles. Screw up your eyes and keep them shut tight. Hold for five seconds then release immediately.

Pause, wait ten seconds, then repeat.

Tense your mouth by clenching your jaws together and concentrate on pressing your lips together as firmly as possible. At the same time you will notice that you tense your eyes. Hold for five seconds then release immediately.

Pause, wait ten seconds, then repeat.

Now concentrate on tensing your neck. Push your chin down a little towards your chest, but do not touch your chest. Hold for five seconds, then release immediately.

Pause, wait ten seconds, then repeat.

Next, move to your shoulders and back, pushing your shoulders up slightly and tensing your neck. Feel the muscles tighten across your shoulders. Hold for five seconds then release immediately.

Pause, wait ten seconds, then repeat.

Tense your shoulders and arms by pushing your arms down, holding your neck rigid. Concentrate on tensing across your shoulders. Hold for five seconds then release immediately.

Pause, wait ten seconds, then repeat.

Tense the muscles in your back by pushing your elbows into your sides, pulling your shoulders down, holding your neck tight and pushing your head down towards your chest and concentrate on tensing the muscles across your back. Hold for five seconds then release immediately.

Pause, wait ten seconds, then repeat.

Now move to your chest and abdomen. Tense the muscles of your chest by pushing your shoulders back, pushing your elbows down into your waist and tilting your head back slightly and concentrate on holding your chest in a barrel-like rigid way. Hold for five seconds then release immediately.

Pause, wait ten seconds, then repeat.

Tense the muscles of your stomach from the back and pull in towards your navel. Hold for five seconds then release immediately.

Pause, wait ten seconds, then repeat.

Next, move to your lower body and legs. Tense your thighs and buttocks by pushing your buttocks down and concentrate on tensing your thighs and buttocks together. Hold for five seconds then release immediately.

Pause, wait ten seconds, then repeat.

Tense your right calf by pulling your toes up towards you, keeping your leg straight at the knee. Pull your toes back until you can feel the pull all the way up your calf muscles. Hold for five seconds then release immediately.

Pause, wait ten seconds, then repeat.

Tense your right foot by curling over your toes, trying to make your toes clench like a first. Hold for five seconds then release immediately.

Pause, wait ten seconds, then repeat.

Repeat this sequence for your left calf and foot.

When you come to this point, begin to tense your whole body, starting with your hands, working up through your arms, then head, neck, shoulders, back, chest, stomach, buttocks, thighs, calves and feet. Take ten seconds to gradually tense the whole body. Hold for five seconds then relax.

As you relax, breathe out as much as you can, slowly. Keep your eyes closed and say 'calm' to yourself.

Repeat this sequence five times, remembering to leave ten seconds between each.

Next, concentrate on slowing down your breathing. Try to fill all your chest and, as you breathe out, say the word 'calm' to yourself. Let your breathing settle into a natural rhythm and then try to fix your mind on a quiet and relaxing scene. Imagine yourself lying on beach or in a meadow. Imagine a warm atmosphere around you. Try to imagine the smells of this environment. Keep your mind as fixed on this place as possible and let yourself drift as much as you can. Don't worry if you fall asleep, but perhaps it may be worth setting your alarm clock first!

Alcohol

Alcohol is the most widely used drug in our society and, for many, the effects are very pleasant and, indeed, beneficial.

It is often used as an instant solution to anxiety, but, if used to excess, alcohol will make your anxiety much worse and lead to a terrible vicious circle. Research has shown that up to 20 per cent of people with agoraphobia may be using alcohol at dangerously high levels. Some surveys have shown that as many as one in three people admitted to alcohol treatment facilities also have a problem with phobias or panic.

Answer the following questions about your drinking habits.

- Do you drink every day?
- Has your tolerance of alcohol changed? Are you drinking more than before to get the same effect?
- Has your capacity for alcohol increased or decreased?
- Do you feel guilty because of your drinking?
- Do you have memory gaps?
- Do friends comment on the amount you drink?
- Do you sometimes feel shaky after a heavy drinking session?
- Do you exceed the safe drinking limit?

There is some controversy over exactly how much is a safe drinking limit. A rough guide, though, and according to current government advice, is that it is safe to drink between 20 and 30 units a week for a man and 15 to 20 units for a woman. A unit is half a pint of beer, a pub measure of spirits or a small (125-ml) glass of 9 per cent strength wine. A very useful website is <www.at-bristol.org.uk/Alcoholandyou/Facts/units.html> as it has a great deal of information.

Although this topic can be controversial, there is little doubt that people who consume more than the safe limits quoted above have a statistically greater chance of developing health problems or suffering social or legal consequences of their drinking (such as relationship problems and driving bans) than those who stick to the limits or drink less.

If you answered 'yes' to any of the above questions, you really need to think about modifying your drinking. One of the great difficulties with answering the questions honestly is that those who have, or who may be developing, an alcohol problem often rationalize their circumstances. They may say, 'I wouldn't drink as much if my boss was nicer to me', 'Anyone would drink if they had my pressures' or 'I have to drink to help me cope with my problem or my anxiety/depression'.

There are some important principles you can follow that will help to ensure your drinking remains enjoyable and without problematic consequences. They are as follows.

- Give yourself an allowance, not exceeding 20 units per week if you are a man, 15 units if you are a woman.
- Always aim to have at least two to three alcohol-free days in any one week and, once or twice a year, give up alcohol for a week or two. Lent is a good time for some.
- Space your drinks. Try to ensure that you never consume more than one unit per half an hour. If you are at a wedding or party that goes on for several hours, do this by drinking non-alcoholic drinks in between or dilute your wine with mineral water or your beer with lemonade.
- Never drink alone.
- Unless it is a social event that is out of the ordinary, never drink during the day.
- Do not drink during working hours.

Try to apply these principles seriously. Use a diary to record your drinking and do this as honestly and accurately as you can. If after three months you are still answering 'yes' to the questions above, you should certainly seek medical advice or go to one of the local alcohol advisory centres. In more severe cases, it may be that you need the help of Alcoholics Anonymous. You can either visit its website – at <www.alcoholics-anonymous.org.uk> – or the address of your local AA group can be found at your GP's surgery, library or in the telephone book.

Diet

It is not uncommon for those who have panic attacks to eat badly, but a hurried eating pattern and an unbalanced diet may actually make your problem worse.

For someone who is already under stress, problems can be

compounded by the intake of high quantities of fat or refined sugar as they may lead to rapid variations in blood sugar. Indeed, it has been known for many years that some people who experience panic attacks may be prone to dips in blood sugar levels (hypoglycaemia), which may, in turn, lead to further anxiety.

Some people with anxiety states also hurry their meals, thus causing physical symptoms and long-term digestive problems. It is, therefore, worth considering following the advice given below.

- Remember to take plenty of time to enjoy your meals – try not to rush them. Allow yourself at least 30 minutes to eat a meal.
- Reduce the speed at which you eat. Put your knife and fork down between mouthfuls, concentrating instead on chewing and enjoying the taste.
- Eat plenty of carbohydrates – pasta, bread, rice and potatoes.
- Ensure that your diet contains sufficient fibre – this will help you to feel satisfied for longer. Eat unrefined carbohydrates, such as wholemeal or granary bread, eat potatoes with their skins left on, eat beans and pulses and have dried and fresh fruits as snacks.
- Avoid refined foods, such as sugar, white bread and fast foods.
- Eat five portions of fresh fruit and vegetables every day.
- Reduce your fat intake – grill foods rather than fry them, use skimmed rather than full-fat milk and substitute low-fat cheeses for full-fat varieties or else eat full-fat cheeses only once or twice a week.
- Try to eat three or four meals a day, making sure that you start with a good breakfast – fruit and cereal are good!
- Avoid snacks but, if you must, eat fruit and vegetables (dried, frozen or fresh).
- Eat with a companion if you can.
- Don't eat your last meal too late at night and try, if possible, to take a gentle walk after you have eaten.

Omega 3

Over the past 20 years, research into the metabolism of the brain has demonstrated that a number of essential fatty acids called Omega 3 seem to be associated with better mental health.

These fatty acids are found in fish and it has been noted that in communities which consume fish in high quantities there is a lower overall incidence of mental illness. Omega 3 is made up of substances that are responsible for the healthy functioning of membranes in the brain and body.

The benefits of Omega 3 to cardiac health have been known about for many years. An increasing amount of evidence now demonstrates that it also seems to benefit people who suffer from depression and schizophrenia. Indeed, a number of studies have demonstrated this, leading many psychiatrists to advocate Omega 3 as a treatment for depression.

One of the leading researchers in this area is Professor Basant Puri, who works at the University of London. He has identified an important component of Omega 3, known as EPA. Furthermore, he has stated that EPA needs to be provided in a special form called ethyl EPA. For more information, read Puri and Boyd's book, *The Natural Way to Beat Depression: The groundbreaking discovery of EPA to change your life.*

Ethyl EPA is available as an over-the-counter supplement called Veg EPA, which is completely free of any of the toxins that contaminate ordinary fish oils.

The evidence concerning the link between EPA and good mental health is very clear. Logically, it follows that people with anxiety disorders might also derive benefit from taking such a supplement. There is plentiful evidence that taking a supplement of Omega 3 in reasonable doses does no harm, so, as it might also do a great deal of good, it is well worth trying it out. Note, however, that research into the use of Omega 3 to treat anxiety disorders still needs to be carried out.

Time management

Many people with anxiety states feel great pressure and urgency and may have high levels of irritability and anger. They often seem to be attempting to do more than is realistic and are forever trying to put a proverbial quart into a pint pot. This pattern obviously leads to very high levels of stress.

There are several principles that you should follow to ensure that you manage your time more effectively.

- Set yourself reasonable and attainable goals. Set ones for the short, medium and long term. Accept, however, that some of your goals may not be attained.
- Ensure that your goals cover all areas of your life, not just work or household duties. Remember to include your hobbies and personal interests.
- Set daily and weekly priorities. Try to list all the things that you want to do in a week and then decide which are the most important.

Remember that we can never achieve all that we want to achieve. Be reasonable and realistic about the priorities you set for yourself.

• Set aside a reasonable amount of time for each activity and allow for unexpected interruptions. Try to plan each day so that you work on your priorities, but remember that life often throws up unexpected interruptions. Some flexibility is, therefore, required.

Time management is based on such simple commonsense principles. The first major element is recognizing that you may put too much pressure on yourself. Most people with time management problems are pressured by themselves rather than others. Taking the pressure off yourself will help you to feel more relaxed so that, in the long run, your susceptibility to anxiety will be decreased.

10

Evaluating your progress

How do you know that you are improving? There are several inventories, questionnaires and rating scales that may be used to measure your level of phobia or panic. These usually involve rating how much anxiety you feel in a specific situation or recording your thoughts or reactions to certain objects or situations.

In my view, although such rating scales, questionnaires and inventories may be very helpful for a professional therapist, they are less helpful for the person in question. The most reliable way to evaluate your progress is to use your problem and target definitions, sit down with a friend, partner or spouse (or cotherapist) and decide how much progress you have made towards your targets.

Furthermore, a simple recording of your day-to-day behaviour in a diary is the final arbiter of success. Simply put, if you have a phobia and have managed to face the object or situation increasingly often and with decreasing levels of anxiety, you are getting better. If you are still avoiding it, you are not making progress.

The examples of diaries on pp. 78–9 showed an anxiety scale, ranging from 0 to 8, to help you record the strength of your feelings of anxiety. Changes in these scores over time also enable you to see how you have progressed. You should not expect your anxiety ratings to drop dramatically when you start a self-help programme, but, if you are facing the phobic situation regularly, they should gradually reduce. For example, you might move from a 7 to a 6, 6 to a 5 and so on as a result of exposure to the phobic object or situation. As you progress, the amount of time it takes to feel each reduction in anxiety should also lessen. There will, however, always be exceptions to this, so do not be worried if you experience an occasional surge in anxiety or if you have an occasional few instances of exposure where your anxiety level remains high.

If after, say, ten exposures there is no real reduction in your anxiety, you need to think again about whether or not these sessions are being properly carried out. One common reason for failing to make progress is that your sessions are not long enough. Lengthening the time you spend exposing yourself to the feared object or situation is the first obvious strategy to improving your progress.

There are, however, other reasons for lack of progress and occasionally one hears of people who make progress with some aspects of their problems, but not others. If this is the case, simply change the focus of your exposure, perhaps concentrating for a while on those parts of your plan that are more successful and returning to the more difficult part(s) when you have had more success.

It is also worthwhile discussing progress with your cotherapist or, if you are a member of a self-help organization, with your contact there. This is often helpful. Although setting yourself exposure tasks is a simple procedure, it can sometimes be very beneficial to have somebody outside the situation give some objective comments.

If you haven't been keeping a diary, take another look at pp. 78–9, work through the points on defining your problem and deciding what your targets are, then, using the examples provided, draw up a diary that is suitable for you.

Conclusion

At this point, you need to evaluate your progress by looking at your original targets. Take each in turn and assess what progress you have made. Don't worry too much if you are doing better in some areas than others. If there is a particular sticking point, leave it alone for a while and return to it later.

You should expect some improvement in your anxiety ratings, but assume that progress may be slow and there will be occasions when you will experience setbacks.

The central message here is that you must persist with your exposure sessions and try to keep to your plan. Don't be afraid to reconsider your list of problems and targets (with the help of your cotherapist if appropriate) and adjust your plan: then take the appropriate action.

11

You really can do it!

Fears and phobias are, in my opinion, an integral part of the human condition. In the UK, the number of people who have fears and phobias, at a level that causes upset to everyday life, is not thousands or hundreds of thousands but millions. It is therefore clear that it will never be possible to provide professional help for all these people, even if we had the most utopian of healthcare systems.

Having said that, it is also clear to me, after 30-something years working in the field, many people have anxiety problems, but, for whatever reason, do not want to be treated by a professional. In my opinion, for these people and others, self-help is a greatly underrated method for dealing with fears and phobias. There is an increasing amount of research evidence that has concluded, for some people, self-help is as effective or even more effective than professional interventions delivered by highly trained individuals.

I appreciate that not all of the suggestions given in this book will suit all those with fears and phobias. If that is the case for you, I would suggest you identify those parts of the book you have found to be helpful and concentrate on those sections. One thing it is crucial to remember, though, is that exposure to what you fear is a non-negotiable precondition for overcoming your fears and phobias. Call this exposure what you may – desensitization, flooding or simply facing your fears – it should be central to whatever you do. I appreciate that facing your fears and phobias will usually involve a measure of anxiety and distress, but the old maxim 'No pain, no gain' is true for the vast majority of people who embark on a programme of either self-help or professional treatment.

Contrary to the message sometimes given by health professionals that six or ten sessions will 'cure' a problem, some people need months or even years to overcome their difficulties. I think I learned this lesson most acutely during the late 1980s when I assisted many people with anxiety problems to taper off their benzodiazepine (Valium-like) tranquillizers. They often took a year or more to withdraw from their medication and then another year or more to overcome the fears that had been the original reason for being prescribed these drugs.

One of the most important lessons I have learned is that each person with a fear or a phobia is different from the next. There is no formula for any problem; everyone is different. There is certainly no magic formula for recovery either. One of the most important things in my professional life, however, has been the satisfaction that I have derived from seeing people overcome sometimes apparently insurmountable levels of fear and anxiety. Whatever your fears or phobias may be, you must know one simple truth: there is every reason to hope that you, too, will overcome them.

Useful contacts

Alcoholics Anonymous
Tel.: 01904 644026
National Helpline: 0845 769 7555
Website: www.alcoholics-anonymous.org.uk

A worldwide organization with groups all over the UK, meeting seven days a week (the website provides local contact information).

Beat the Benzos
Tel.: 01457 876355
Website: www.benzo.org.uk/btb2.htm

This organization campaigns for better services for those dependent on benzodiazepine drugs, such as diazepam (Valium). It also offers information and local support groups.

British Association for Behavioural and Cognitive Psychotherapies
Tel.: 0161 797 4484
Website: www.babcp.com

This multidisciplinary organization is not only the main interest group for those interested in behavioural and cognitive psychotherapy, but BABCP also provides accreditation for those who have received appropriate training and who are in receipt of appropriate levels of supervision and continuing professional development. It is recognized by employers within the NHS and independent sector, as well as by the private health insurers. BABCP provides national and international conferences and local workshops on specific topics.

British Psychological Society
Tel.: 0116 254 9568
Website: www.bps.org.uk

The website includes a helpful 'Find a psychologist' search facility and a register of chartered psychologists.

Mind
Tel.: 020 8519 2122
Mind*info*Line: 0845 766 0163
Website: www.mind.org.uk

Mind is the UK's leading mental health charity. The organization provides considerable information about mental health problems and local resources.

Mind Cymru (Wales)
Tel.: 029 2039 5123

NHS Direct
Tel.: 0845 4647
Website: www.nhsdirect.nhs.uk

NHS Direct provides information about health, illness and health services to enable people to make decisions about their own health care and that of their family.

No Panic
Tel.: 01952 590005
Freephone Helpline: 0808 808 0545 (10 a.m.–10 p.m., every day; ring 0044 1952 590545 from outside the UK)
Website: www.nopanic.org.uk

This is the largest self-help organization for people with anxiety disorders in the UK and Republic of Ireland, and provides a wide range of written literature, as well as a telephone helpline and telephone recovery groups run by people who have experienced anxiety disorders. These telephone recovery groups are based on cognitive behavioural principles.

No Panic Ireland
Tel.: 01 272 1872
Helpline: 01 272 1897 (10 a.m.–1 p.m. and 7–10 p.m., Monday to Friday)
Website: www.nopanic.org.uk/npireland2.htm

The No Panic Ireland helpline was launched in August 2004 and took in excess of 1500 calls in its first year. It is now staffed by Irish volunteers.

OCD Action
Tel.: 0845 390 6232 or 020 7253 2664
Website: www.ocdaction.org.uk/obsessive-compulsive-disorder

OCD Action is the leading national charity for people with obsessive–compulsive disorder (OCD) and related conditions. It provides a very wide range of information, offers local support groups for people with OCD and their families, and supports a range of research activities.

Samaritans
Tel.: 08457 909090
Website: www.samaritans.org

Samaritans is one of the UK's most respected charities. It offers confidential support to people experiencing a crisis or thinking of taking their own lives or of harming themselves.

Self Help UK
Website: www.self-help.org.uk

Self Help UK is a free service that provides information on over 1000 self-help organizations, patient support groups and charities across the UK. These provide support, guidance and advice to patients, their carers and their relatives. The groups and organizations that are covered embrace many medical conditions, diseases and treatments.

Triumph over Phobia
Tel.: 0845 600 9601
Website: www.topuk.org

Triumph over Phobia (TOP UK) is a UK-registered charity which aims to help people with phobias, obsessive–compulsive disorder and related anxiety disorders to overcome their fears. It achieves this by running a network of self-help therapy groups. Groups meet weekly and are structured, warm and supportive.

NICE guidelines

These clinical guidelines provide all the reader needs to know about the assessment, management and treatment of the conditions listed on the next page. The NICE website (<www.nice.org.uk>) provides, for each of these guidelines, a very wide range of downloadable materials, from lay summaries for the general public, to quick reference guides for busy clinicians, to the full guidelines, which contain numerous references.

Anxiety
Website: www.nice.org.uk/guidance/CG22

Clinical guidelines CG22 (issued December 2004). Management of anxiety (panic disorder, with or without agoraphobia, and generalized anxiety disorder) in adults in primary, secondary and community care.

Obsessive–compulsive disorder and body dysmorphic disorder
Website: www.nice.org.uk/guidance/CG31

Clinical guidelines CG31 (issued November 2005).

Post-traumatic stress disorder
Website: www.nice.org.uk/guidance/CG26

Clinical guidelines CG26 (issued March 2005).

Relaxation exercises

Breathing exercises and relaxation instructions
Website: www.ntu.ac.uk/sss/self_help/14105gp.html

Deep muscle relaxation exercises
Website: www.aleph1.co.uk/stress-management-biofeedback

Video clip: breathing exercises for panic
Website: www.panicattackcorner.com/panic-attack-videos/how-to-alleviate-panic-attacks-how-to-do-breathing-exercises.htm

References

Brown, G. and Harris, T. (1978) *Social Origins of Depression*, London, Tavistock.

Herbert, Dr Claudia (2002) *Understanding Your Reactions to Trauma: A guide for survivors of trauma and their families* (revised edition), Oxford, Blue Stallion Publications, Oxford.
A very informative guide that I always suggest people with trauma-related problems read before embarking on a treatment programme. It contains very useful advice on managing symptoms.

Marks, I. M. (1987) *Fears, Phobias and Rituals*, Oxford, Oxford University Press.
This is a definitive text that describes every aspect of fears, phobias and rituals and remains the best source of background information. There is no other book that comprehensively addresses the background research and, although more than two decades have passed since the book was published, much of the material still holds true. You should be aware, however, that you will need to update your knowledge on the treatment approaches mentioned.

Marks, I. M. (2005) *Living with Fear*, Maidenhead, McGraw-Hill.
A new edition of the original self-help book for phobias and still a good read after over 30 years!

Phillips, K. (2005) *Broken Mirror: Understanding and treating body dysmorphic disorder*, New York, Oxford University Press.
This is a comprehensive but very readable account of body dysmorphic disorder, written by the USA's leading expert on this condition. Although it is now slightly dated, it is perhaps the best book to recommend to someone who has this condition and, used in conjunction with NICE's guidelines, is also an excellent source of reference for practitioners.

Puri, B. H. and Boyd, H. (2004) *The Natural Way to Beat Depression: The groundbreaking discovery of EPA to change your life*, London, Hodder Mobius.

Veale, D. and Willson, R. (2006) *Overcoming Obsessive Compulsive Disorder: A self-help guide using cognitive behavioural techniques*, London, Robinson.
This book is not only a most comprehensive self-help manual but also a source of up-to-date information and evidence. As well as recommending this book to those with this disorder, mental health professionals will also find this to be an excellent source of information.

Veale, D. and Willson, R. (2009) *Overcoming Body Image Problems Including Body Dysmorphic Disorder: A self-help guide using cognitive behavioural techniques*, London, Robinson.
This is the only self-help book for this disorder. It was written by a psychiatrist and a psychologist who conducted the first research (with myself) into the disorder in the UK.

Willson, R. and Branch, R. (2005) *Cognitive Behavioural Therapy for Dummies*, London, John Wiley.
The title is somewhat misleading, as this is certainly not dumbed down. The book is probably the best comprehensive guide to cognitive behaviour therapy for people who are contemplating this form of treatment and it serves as a very useful adjunct to professional help. One of the most useful things about the book is that it provides very clear accounts of lots of techniques that can be used to great effect when dealing with some of the problems associated with anxiety disorders. It is also very useful to therapists during their training.

Index

111